Essential Business Fundamentals for the Successful Eye Care Practice

Savak Teymoorian, MD, MBA
Cataract and Glaucoma Specialist
Harvard Eye Associates
Laguna Hills, California

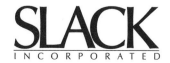

SLACK
INCORPORATED

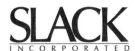

SLACK Incorporated
6900 Grove Road
Thorofare, NJ 08086 USA
856-848-1000   Fax: 856-848-6091
www.Healio.com/books
© 2019 by SLACK Incorporated

Senior Vice President: Stephanie Arasim Portnoy
Vice President, Editorial: Jennifer Kilpatrick
Vice President, Marketing: Michelle Gatt
Acquisitions Editor: Tony Schiavo
Managing Editor: Allegra Tiver
Creative Director: Thomas Cavallaro
Cover Artist: Anita Santiago
Project Editor: Joseph Lowery

Dr. Savak Teymoorian is a consultant for Aerie, Alcon, Allergan, Bausch + Lomb, Ellex, Glaukos, Ivantis, MDbackline. com, New World Medical, and Omeros. He has done research for Aerie, Allergan, Bausch + Lomb, and Glaukos. He also receives royalties from SLACK Incorporated and is a speaker for Allergan, Bausch + Lomb, Ellex, and Glaukos.

The procedures and practices described in this publication should be implemented in a manner consistent with the professional standards set for the circumstances that apply in each specific situation. Every effort has been made to confirm the accuracy of the information presented and to correctly relate generally accepted practices. The authors, editors, and publisher cannot accept responsibility for errors or exclusions or for the outcome of the material presented herein. There is no expressed or implied warranty of this book or information imparted by it. Care has been taken to ensure that drug selection and dosages are in accordance with currently accepted/recommended practice. Off-label uses of drugs may be discussed. Due to continuing research, changes in government policy and regulations, and various effects of drug reactions and interactions, it is recommended that the reader carefully review all materials and literature provided for each drug, especially those that are new or not frequently used. Some drugs or devices in this publication have clearance for use in a restricted research setting by the Food and Drug and Administration or FDA. Each professional should determine the FDA status of any drug or device prior to use in their practice.

Any review or mention of specific companies or products is not intended as an endorsement by the author or publisher.

SLACK Incorporated uses a review process to evaluate submitted material. Prior to publication, educators or clinicians provide important feedback on the content that we publish. We welcome feedback on this work.

Library of Congress Cataloging-in-Publication Data

Names: Teymoorian, Savak, author.
Title: Essential business fundamentals for the successful eye care practice /
 Savak Teymoorian.
Description: Thorofare, NJ : SLACK Incorporated, [2018] | Includes
 bibliographical references and index.
Identifiers: LCCN 2018023130 (print) | LCCN 2018023999 (ebook) | ISBN
 9781630914066 (Epub) | ISBN 9781630914073 (Web) | ISBN 9781630914059 (pbk.
 : alk. paper)
Subjects: | MESH: Optometry--organization & administration | Practice
 Management
Classification: LCC RE959.3 (ebook) | LCC RE959.3 (print) | NLM WW 704 | DDC
 617.7/5068--dc23
LC record available at https://lccn.loc.gov/2018023130

Printed in the United States of America.

Last digit is print number: 10   9   8   7   6   5   4   3   2   1

Dedication

To my Lord and Savior, Jesus Christ, for being my Hero.
To Sarah and Samantha for your endless love, support, and encouragement.
To Haidook and Aras for showing me the real meaning of sacrifice.
To Mark and Pam for taking me in as one of your own.
To Silano for always being my buddy.

CONTENTS

ACKNOWLEDGMENTS

Numerous individuals have inspired, supported, and encouraged me along the journey of writing this book. In particular, I would like to acknowledge Arsen Grigoryan, MBA. A sincere thank you for your time and assistance in helping to complete this project.

A special thanks to my partners, associates, and staff at Harvard Eye Associates. I appreciate the trust and belief from Dr. Roger Ohanesian, Dr. Edward Kim, Dr. Diana Kersten, Dr. John Hovanesian, Dr. Chuck Keller, Dr. Brian Kim, Dr. Duna Raoof, Dr. Jeff Jacobs, Dr. Nicki Stefanidis, Dr. Karen Skvarna, and Dr. Mark Levy. My actual experience in the business of medicine would not have occurred without their support and patience.

I also want to acknowledge the care and training I received during my glaucoma fellowship at Stanford University's Byers Eye Institute. This includes the exceptional teachings of Dr. Kuldev Singh and Dr. Robert Chang along with the warm and friendly hospitality of the ancillary staff. The nurturing atmosphere they created was critical to my development.

I still owe a lot of gratitude to the Department of Ophthalmology at the University of Missouri, Kansas City. It was with their belief in me that I received the opportunity to pursue my lifelong goal of being an ophthalmologist. I simply cannot express how grateful I am for that chance. I would like to thank all the faculty and staff that dedicated their valuable time to train me. I consider them my extended family. The following individuals taught me special lessons in business that I want to note: Dr. Felix Sabates for the persistence needed to be successful, Dr. Nelson Sabates for the demonstration of leadership and all-around business acumen, Dr. Jean Hausheer for the skills to encourage and manage others, Dr. Michael Cassell for the weekly business sessions and the belief I could accomplish anything in ophthalmology, and Mrs. Saundra Thompson for being the glue that kept us together.

I want to recognize all my coresidents with a special thanks to Vinay, Ashley, Erica, Ryan, Brian, Ken, Bill, Florin, Mou, Jessica, Shamim, Nick, Luke, and Adam for allowing me to both lead and follow them. I hope you learned as much from me as I did from you. I celebrate in your accomplishments and look forward to seeing what is ahead of us.

I need to especially acknowledge the faculty and staff at the University of California, Irvine School of Medicine and the Paul Merage School of Business. These 2 programs are responsible for the unique skill set I possess due to my MD/MBA training. The foundation for my entire career and this book derives from that education. I hope to share their teachings with all of my readers.

Lastly, many thanks to SLACK Incorporated for its commitment and shared vision on the value of this book's topic. I especially want to highlight Tony Schiavo, whose guidance and support has been monumental along the way. I also would like to show my appreciation to Stephanie Portnoy and Jennifer Kilpatrick for their time and effort.

My sincere hope is that everyone that has influenced the writing of this book understands what a significant, positive impact it has made on taking care of other people. When doctors are better trained, especially in areas of limited education and exposure, patients benefit.

— Sev

ABOUT THE AUTHOR

Savak "Sev" Teymoorian, MD, MBA grew up in Southern California. He attended Glendale High School and completed his undergraduate studies at the University of California, Irvine. He graduated Magna Cum Laude with a Bachelor's Degree in the Biological Sciences and a Focus in the Neurosciences. He remained at UC Irvine following his acceptance into the competitive MD/MBA program, a unique collaboration between the School of Medicine and the Paul Merage School of Business.

Dr. Teymoorian and his wife Sarah, who is also a physician, moved to Kansas City after fulfilling his internship commitment in Internal Medicine at UC Irvine. He completed his residency training in ophthalmology at the University of Missouri, Kansas City. In his last year, the department faculty honored him with the selection to serve as Chief Resident. His training continued with an advanced fellowship in glaucoma at Stanford University.

Dr. Teymoorian and his family then moved back to Orange County, California. He is currently a partner at Harvard Eye Associates, a large, multi-specialty private practice with multiple locations throughout the region. He focuses primarily on glaucoma and cataract surgery. Dr. Teymoorian is actively involved in ophthalmology clinical research for both medical and surgical glaucoma therapy. He also participates in mission trips abroad to provide ocular treatment to those without access to it.

As a key opinion leader, Dr. Teymoorian has been invited to present at numerous conferences over a wide range of topics given his unique skill set and experience. By living and working in Orange County, he actively collaborates with industry leaders to advance the field of eye care. He frequently contributes to articles in literature and print magazines. He actively maintains a blog for *Ocular Surgery News* that discusses a broad range of topics about the entire glaucoma landscape. With the growing demand of teaching medical professionals about business, Dr. Teymoorian complements the topics discussed in this book with additional resources available on his website listed below.

Dr. Teymoorian enjoys spending his spare time with Sarah and their daughter, Samantha. They like visiting nearby beaches and traveling to new destinations. The family can be found both taking part in and watching sporting activities. They also actively attend Saddleback Church.

Website: www.drteymoorian.com
Twitter: @DrTeymoorian

FOREWORD

The training required to practice medicine is long and arduous. It starts with the study of theory and eventually moves to guided practice via residencies and fellowships. Once physicians have gained the requisite medical knowledge and experience, they are thrown into the business world of practicing medicine.

For those who choose to go into private practice, they are miraculously expected to negotiate contracts with a new employer; become responsible for accounts receivable; deal with human resources; obey the patchwork of laws that govern HR, OSHA, and HIPAA; become an expert coder with insurance claims; and a lot more. Our medical training does not help us here; we are forced to find our way through this unfamiliar business maze while we see patients, perform surgery, stay current with our respective subspecialty fields and network to grow the practice. Essentially, we are tossed into the business world with our hands handcuffed behind us.

Savak Teymoorian, MD, MBA has made a great contribution to balance our lopsided education with *Essential Business Fundamentals for the Successful Eye Care Practice*. He noticed the anxiety and frustration among many of his colleagues who entered private practice. Despite being highly trained physicians, it was clear that they lacked the business skill set to navigate the unfamiliar landscape. To fill this void, Dr. Teymoorian shares his secrets by distilling the essential business fundamentals and succinctly presents them in a format familiar to physicians.

In *Essential Business Fundamentals for the Successful Eye Care Practice*, Dr. Teymoorian shares his insights on the difference between a leader and a manager. He outlines how to create an organizational culture through key administrative and financial models for successful patient care.

Dr. Teymoorian's book is a must-read for every physician whether just coming out of fellowship or in practice for years. It provides the necessary bridge from medical training to running a successful, patient-centric medical business.

Cynthia Matossian, MD, FACS
Clinical Assistant Professor of Ophthalmology (Adjunct)
Temple University School of Medicine
Philadelphia, Pennsylvania

INTRODUCTION

You can never cross the ocean until you have the courage to lose sight of the shore.
—Christopher Columbus

This journey into business will make you feel uncomfortable, and that's a good thing. The adventure is worth it. The usual reaction from most eye care practitioners, both ophthalmologists and optometrists, is one of apprehension and nervousness when presented with business-related issues. Think back to your first day of graduate training. Is it fair to say there were similar feelings of discomfort? You were presented with a mountain of information about something you only knew superficially. Then, after receiving a fundamentally sound education, the very complex organ of the eye became second nature.

How did that happen? It is like every other difficult challenge you faced in life. You stepped out of the comfort zone and allowed yourself to be vulnerable to make some mistakes. You arrived at your new destination a much-improved person through hard work and persistence. To all of my eye care practitioner colleagues, the process of learning business is the same way. Not only is it possible for you to understand business, but also to excel in it. The only reason you feel uneasy in this area is that you were never given a chance to learn it in school. It is difficult to construct a beautiful skyscraper without a sturdy foundation. My hope is that this book provides the necessary groundwork that will enable future success in your business.

The real world expects us to be proficient in both ocular medicine and business regardless of what was included in our respective graduate training. Everyone agrees if a patient has a medical issue, then the doctor should address it; however, the provider also hears about nonmedical problems. A patient can complain to the doctor about a bad experience he or she had with the front office staff; one employee may mention she needs a raise while another implies he feels harassed at work; a creditor can leave a phone message regarding the late payment on a loan for a piece of equipment that was purchased; and a government official could walk into the office wanting to know what the office does to ensure patient confidentiality. However, we were never given the lessons or provided the thought process on how to respond when faced with these business problems. You may have even wanted to pursue an MBA to learn more about business but never had the time to do it.

There is a silver lining to this predicament. Your ability to be accepted into and successfully complete advanced ocular training can be transferred to the field of business. You have proven to possess the required skill set to quickly process essential information and apply it to practice. All that is needed are the fundamental tools to get you there. First, you must have the courage to admit your deficiencies; and second, you need to open your mind to learn new areas of knowledge beyond medicine. This is why I am excited to share with you what I acquired in MBA training, but present it in the way I learned best during my MD education. The intention is to succinctly deliver the needed information through a very familiar, efficient presentation to maximize your knowledge, while minimizing the required time to obtain it.

This book is divided into chapters with each one focusing on an important business topic. The introduction at the beginning summarizes the essential information discussed in the text. The rest of the chapter divides into the same 4 sections throughout the book. The initial section provides a fundamental understanding of what the section is about and how it relates to business. The next portion subdivides into 3 parts. The first discusses why this area is important for any provider. The second part outlines and defines the critical words, phrases, and principles within that space. The third portion integrates the prior sections by providing real life applications of these business topics that we commonly face in our medical practice. The last section poses specific, thought-provoking questions that will direct you to meaningful action items that can be executed at your work today. After each chapter, critical take-home points are offered as a quick-reference guide for the future.

The reader will notice that the material from the chapters is intertwined and complementary. Like the organs in the human body, these topics cannot work independently. They rely on mutually beneficial relationships that help one another function well. The ability to integrate these discrete subjects into one unit produces a synergistic outcome that has greater value than its individual pieces.

It is also important to take a moment to understand what this book is not. This style of text is written to provide the absolute essentials in each of these key business areas. Therefore, it is not meant to offer a masterly level of subject coverage. The goal is for the reader to become familiar with the key words and principles that drive discussions and decisions in business. It is meant to unlock the sealed doors to business by learning the necessary vocabulary terms. This is the same process that occurs in medicine. For example, it's like the "aha" moment for the young practitioner that finally understands the meaning of proliferative diabetic retinopathy with macular edema. The book should leave the reader with the foundation to actively participate in business activities. This includes recognizing when things do not look right and requesting clarification from those managing it. As a note, professional help should always be sought after if more information is needed.

The primary intended audience for this book are eye care practitioners: ophthalmologists and optometrists. However, it will become evident that the lessons taught are applicable to any type of doctor or staff in the medical field. This extends to the various work environments beyond private practice. You will encounter the use of many words to identify the individual and describe the structure in which he or she provides care. The application of this text goes beyond the initial targeted reader. Please share it with those who you think would also benefit. As you will soon see, this behavior of considering and improving others is an example of great leadership.

At the culmination of this book and its journey, my personal goal is that you feel at home in this new neighborhood of business. I measure my success on your willingness to settle down and enthusiastically set up shop in a place where you were once anxious to visit. Your new address: the very desirable property at the intersection of Eye Care Street and Business Avenue. Now, let's join hands and experience this adventure together.

1

Providing Leadership

If your actions inspire others to dream more, learn more,
do more and become more, you are a leader.

— John Quincy Adams

INTRODUCTION

The title of *Doctor* places many responsibilities on an individual. Some of these are obvious while others are not quite as clear. The role of *leader* exemplifies the latter. Certain practitioners feel their only job is to provide ocular care, and it has nothing to do with leadership; however, if people feel comfortable enough to place their vision in your hands, they will naturally turn to your leadership at other difficult times, whether you want them to or not. It is an incredible compliment to be thought of that way. The result of this is that your acceptance and ability to effectively lead will impact your company's overall success.

Leadership is simply guiding and influencing others. At the highest level, the practitioner provides direction about an organization's goals and demonstrates its culture. This includes the desired reputation in the community among colleagues and the quality of patient care given to customers. These leadership duties extend to many other tasks such as directing change. If needed, the provider will convert a toxic work environment to one where valuable recruits want to join it. Another example includes developing and training that star low-level technician with jagged edges to eventually become a well-polished office manager.

Although understanding the meaning of leadership is important, the successful eye care practitioner also comprehends how great leadership is executed. Therefore, this chapter begins with a section about key strategic questions that must first be

Teymoorian S. *Essential Business Fundamentals*
for the Successful Eye Care Practice (pp 1-19).
© 2019 SLACK Incorporated.

skillfully addressed. The answers to these provide the company's direction and identity. The attention then shifts to 5 critical leadership activities that promote a winning organization. This chapter aims to help readers recognize how they will be seen as leaders in their organization and motivates them to capitalize on these opportunities to improve themselves and others during the process.

WHAT IS LEADERSHIP?

A plethora of examples exist in history where a business had a valuable product but never became successful. Creating and running a thriving company also requires intangible assets that can be easily taken for granted. The ability to possess and demonstrate leadership is a perfect example. It can even be considered "the secret sauce" that enables an innovative concept to become a reality.

What are the qualities of an excellent leader? Although there are many attributes, one underlying trait is the capability to maximize other people's abilities. A common misconception is that leaders only affect those individuals reporting to them. However, this definition more closely resembles managers. There is an important distinction between managers and leaders. Managers control the activities of those they govern. Leaders are quite different with much broader-reaching results. Their influence is felt throughout the entire business, regardless of who reports to them, now and into the future.[1]

An important display of leadership is affecting the culture of a business. It is the culture that provides the blueprint for the organization's building blocks. It directs 2 critical questions. The first is where it wants to be in the future, or its vision.[2] The second is what it wants to be, or its mission. After these are established, the remaining task is to execute the plan to reach these goals. This includes harnessing the leader's skill set to maximize the organization's human resources by empowering employees to exercise their own leadership.

LEADERSHIP IN EYE CARE

The benefits from leadership are not easily noticed during peaceful times. However, when tensions are high and consequences are meaningful, the presence and ability to effectively lead becomes priceless. It can mean the difference between eventual success or failure of the organization and all of its employees.

Leadership is the glue for businesses that holds all the pieces together and provides the overall mold to create the desired shape. Its extensive reach directs the positioning and executing of all the other arms in a company. This is accomplished by supplying the fundamental principles about the practice's identity and goals. Successful eye care practitioners perform the following: exemplify the culture, form the vision statement, create the mission statement, lead change, develop talent, empower the employees, encourage teamwork, and manage conflict.

Exemplifying the Culture

Importance

One of the most underappreciated but vital activities to build and maintain a prosperous company is the development of the right culture. It is easy to see the problems individuals run into by not realizing the value of an organization's culture. The first association people make when thinking about business is money. Although wealth is important, the financial capabilities of a business are simply the downstream effects of how successfully it is run. The driver for all operations, however, is its culture. The proof to this statement is that culture will play a role in every other chapter of this book.

The culture serves as a compass to direct activities and guide decisions. It supplies the framework for the practice's expectations of employee behavior with each other and customers. To illustrate the fundamental application of culture, consider the common dilemma of how an employee should react when confronted with a problem that does not have a standard response in the company's protocol. The quality of the decisions made at these moments on a day-to-day basis are what separates the best businesses from the rest. If the culture is one of valuing relationships, acting professionally, and providing the best service, then this is how the employee will react in that and any other similar situation. Employees will naturally conduct themselves in a manner and present an answer that is consistent with the company's culture. Unfortunately, this is also true if the culture is defined by less than favorable characteristics.

The takeaway message is that the individuals who influence the culture in an organization play a critical role. They are the true leaders by defining and demonstrating its values. It is imperative to have the right culture that is built upon the company's desired qualities. This circles back to the initial thoughts on how people mistakenly only associate the success of a business with its ability to make money. The thriving eye care practitioner understands that the real force in a winning organization is its culture.

Keywords

Leader: A person that provides leadership

Culture: The long-term image and behavior of an organization that is exemplified by leadership and seen as the appropriate way for employees to conduct themselves

Leadership: The ability to guide and provide influence to others in both an individual and group setting

Influence: The process of affecting the behavior and thoughts of others

Model: The act of exemplifying a quality, behavior, or action

Manager: A person that fills a role designated by a company that controls the activities of a group of employees

Applications

The staff members within an eye care practice look toward their leaders to provide the company's culture and ground rules. These select individuals have the keen leadership abilities to influence others by connecting, encouraging, empowering, and orienting.[1] People are naturally drawn and want to follow these types of human beings. However, this quality places the responsibility to lead well on these individuals. Their words and actions model to everyone else the expected conduct within the organization. The requisite to creating a top culture is having outstanding leaders that exemplify it. On the other hand, leaders with a negative attitude will disseminate and produce an equally poor culture.

Identifying these leaders is not as straightforward as one would assume. Most individuals inaccurately believe a manager or anyone in a supervisory role is a leader, and that only people in high-ranking positions can be leaders. These are misconceptions. Managers are not necessarily leaders, and leaders do not have to be managers. Anyone in any position within an organization can lead. In fact, a sign of a great leader is one that understands how to lead from the middle of an organization. His or her actions can affect those above, below, and at the same level as him- or herself.

How does one lead without having an official managerial title? There are many methods, including some that are easy, of how any employee can create a great culture. For example, consider an associate physician without an ownership stake in a practice. He or she shows leadership by knowing the name of all the staff members and something important about them. This creates a special bond and demonstrates that everyone is appreciated. A simple statement like the following is sometimes worth more than a raise to an employee: "John, thank for your help today working up those last few patients; and, by the way, how did Tommy's Little League baseball game go?"

Leaders are consistent with their words and behaviors. They walk the walk and talk the talk. When these individuals go down a hallway, they lean over to pick up trash on the ground even when no is around to see it. Chances are high that this type of positive behavior will be noted at some point and shared among other employees. These actions, much like their reputations, spread like wildfire in an organization and are quite infectious in nature. Everyone else suddenly follows that lead. It becomes expected that any staff member would have picked up that litter because it is the culture. These demonstrations of culture resonate even louder when done by the respected eye care provider.

Outstanding leadership both empowers those around the leaders and also holds them accountable to their actions and responsibilities. They model professional and trustworthy characteristics, and they expect others to follow that lead. Leaders understand that if they treat others like adults, they will act like adults; but if they treat them like children, they will act like children.[3] They influence others into the right actions.

Leading a group also necessitates guiding many individuals with different backgrounds to work as a team. Leaders know that all it takes is one bad apple, or one good apple that has a lapse in judgment, to gossip and destroy the hard-earned trust among the group. The creation of a safe and positive culture is aided when leaders do not partake in gossiping and let others know not to as well. Again, they treat others as adults and expect adult behavior from them.

Immediate Action Items

Do you know your company's culture? Describe it in one succinct sentence. Are you sure your perception of culture is the same as others in your organization? Take a survey of a select few, yet diverse, employees of how they would define the culture. Do their answers match your thoughts? If they match and it is the desired culture, then continue to demonstrate it through your actions and words as a leader in your practice. If the answers do not match or the consensus response is not what the culture should be, then you have taken the first step in the right direction—you have acknowledged that there needs to be an improvement. Use the lessons learned throughout this book to create and exemplify your new winning culture.

If you do not know the culture, ask yourself what you wish the culture to be. Then, question staff members about what they believe the culture currently is in the practice. If that matches, then the great news is you have a head start in this process! The next goal is to reinforce it by role modeling the correct behavior to sustain it moving forward. However, if it does not match, then this is your opportunity to develop the culture you do want to represent your organization. Integrate the information presented throughout this text to achieve this goal.

Forming the Vision Statement

Importance

A method that leaders incorporate to develop and maintain an organization's culture is to provide direction and set goals of where the business should be in the future. Elite leadership not only aligns the company culture to these goals, but also delineates the required steps needed to achieve the desired outcome. An effective vision statement accomplishes this task by serving as a map. Although it can be done verbally, a written vision statement is powerful because of its permanent nature. It signifies strength, commitment, and confidence.

The vision statement helps orient the organization to its future direction.[4] This includes providing clear endpoints, in addition to milestones, to be accomplished along the way. This strategic approach ensures that the day-to-day staff activities will ultimately lead to the company's favored outcome. It also prevents valuable resources from being wasted. With each daily task, employees should be able to confirm that their work will result in the group getting closer to their shared vision.

Keywords

Vision statement: A statement that describes the direction and goals of a group or organization

Goals: The objectives to be met

Strategies: The purposeful use of actions to achieve a goal

Actions: The coordination of tasks to execute a strategy

Tactics: The tasks that are completed to produce an action

Applications

The practical creation of the vision statement takes a backward approach by identifying the required steps needed to reach the preset goals. Effective leaders take those goals and develop strategies to accomplish them. These strategies are a collection of executed actions that are produced through a series of tactics employed by the staff. The tone of the vision statement should be inspiring to create excitement and a sense of purpose. The following is an example:

> Patients with eye disorders deserve the best quality of life possible for them. The doctors and staff at Teymoorian Eye Associates will meet that challenge by being at the leading edge of innovation in this area. Our organization will help pioneer ground-breaking medical and surgical therapies to not only preserve, but also improve the vision of our patients. We will pave the road for better care in the future. This commitment and dedication will result in the highest level of customer service witnessed in Orange County. It will position Teymoorian Eye Associates as the expert and trustworthy practice to successfully handle the tremendous responsibility of caring for everyone's eyesight.

In this example, one goal is to provide the best customer service. A strategy would be to achieve great refractive outcomes from cataract surgery. The actions taken to execute this strategy would be to utilize the best phacoemulsification platforms during surgery and select the right intraocular lens for each patient. The tactics used to execute these actions would include having the ophthalmologists, optometrists, and ancillary staff obtain additional education on the evolving technology to provide knowledgeable guidance to the patients. This process can then be repeated for each of the desired goals to create a series of plans to successfully reach them.

Immediate Action Items

Does your practice have a written vision statement? How old is the latest version and, more importantly, does it match the current desired endpoint for the future? If so, you are ahead of the curve. The next step is to ensure that all employees, both now and in the future, are clearly aware of it. Utilize your Human Resources to incorporate it throughout the practice. Examples include discussing it when onboarding new staff to help them understand the company's vision or during performance reviews to reinforce the purpose for requested employee behavior modification.

If you do not have one, it is time for some serious self-reflection and determination of what the vision should be for your organization. Think carefully about the desired goals and craft a written statement that inspires your employees to work together to reach them. Do not complete this task by yourself; instead, enlist and empower key staff members through this process. This will not only show your entire organization that you value their thoughts, but also you will have their buy-in to its actual results.

If they helped create the vision statement, then it is their own reputation that is at stake for its quality and execution.

Creating the Mission Statement

Importance

An organization's mission statement complements the vision statement and is equally important in function. Leadership must also transmit a clear message about it to the staff. Instead of thinking about the future as described by the vison statement, the mission statement primarily focuses on the present time. Great leaders utilize it as an opportunity to illustrate what the company is by using values as a focal point. The hope is to develop an intimate connection with individuals, including its customers.

The mission statement presents to customers a sense of who and what the business is in an effective manner. Inherently, customers are looking to have their needs met by requesting a service. In this transaction, they give up their hard-earned money and, as a consequence, they develop a set of expectations that need to be met. This is where the value of organizational transparency becomes advantageous for practices that are properly positioned. A company with a clear vision helps ensure that what the customers are anticipating from the relationship matches what the business plans to provide. The ability to successfully link the expectations of the customers to goals of the company makes for a mutually beneficial relationship and develops trust.

Keywords

Mission statement: A statement that represents the purpose and values of a group or organization

Values: The amount of worth someone places on certain things

Honor: A quality of behaving in a manner consistent with the highest moral code

Integrity: The ability to behave in a manner consistent with an individual's values and morals

Loyalty: A degree of allegiance where an individual maintains commitment despite external forces

Applications

The eye care practice uses the mission statement to describe who it treats, what care it provides, and how it serves. The tone is meant to be factual and unambiguous for all its readers. It expresses the practice's purpose and desired qualities. Although there are many powerful values to incorporate in a statement, effective samples include those that instill a feeling of honor and integrity for the staff to emulate. It provides prospective patients a sense of what they should expect with the hopes of developing loyalty to the company. The following is an example of a mission statement:

At Teymoorian Eye Associates, our patients are the number one priority. We continually strive to serve them with the best possible eye care. This is accomplished through constant education in new topics relating to vision along with dedication to maintain superior clinical and surgical skills. We provide these services with honor and integrity as we humbly assume the responsibility to achieve the best vision for our patients. Our relentless commitment to and endless pursuit of exemplary ocular care hopes to earn their loyalty. Whenever we are in doubt of how to act in a situation, we do what we think is best for our patients as if they were our own family.

Immediate Action Items

Does your company have a written mission statement? Is it updated and do all of your employees know it? If so, then continue emphasizing it when possible. This includes activities that highlight positive staff behavior like "Monthly Kudos Note," where a company email is sent recognizing individual or group actions that align with the organization's mission. The simple act of acknowledgement from a leader has resonating effects that raise the highlighted staff members while motivating all others.

If not, then like the vision statement, it is time to carefully consider what you want the practice to be and the goals it needs to achieve. Again, make sure to involve other individuals to draft a statement that inspires, leads, and challenges employees to achieve the desired outcomes. Once it is written, utilize Human Resources to introduce and reinforce it throughout the lifespan of each employee. Provide positive feedback when staff members demonstrate these qualities, but also incorporate it into retraining for those whose actions do not align with it.

Leading Change

Importance

The thought of change makes most people anxious. People naturally resist it. This is especially true of employees that feel secure in an organization since they are satisfied with the status quo.[5] However, it is uncommon in any area of life to be void of situations that necessitate change. Adjustments will be needed; this is a fact of life and also seen in the business world. Change is inevitable because the competitive landscape is dynamic[6]; however, the way it is handled greatly varies. Its approach will either enable success or allow failure.

The hope when leading change is to anticipate it in advance to allow for strategic planning and execution. The reality is that unexpected events develop, and crises emerge. It is under these stressful times that the ability to provide excellent leadership becomes especially valuable. It should not be a surprise that leading change is one of the hardest challenges a leader can face. Those that do succeed view change differently. Instead of thinking about it in terms of an obstacle to achieving a goal, leaders view it as a stepping stone for improvement. The best organizations have strong leadership that convert the time and effort required during these periods of change into a strategic advantage. They do not waste resources, including time spent on any activity.

Keywords

Flexibility: The ability to change and be dynamic based upon current conditions

Competitive landscape: An analysis that first identifies and understands the competitors in a desired marketplace, and then performs a self-evaluation for strengths and weaknesses to guide positioning for success in that space

Internal environment: The happenings and atmosphere inside an organization

External environment: The happenings and atmosphere outside an organization

Climate: A set of internal, short-term perceptions of individuals about an organization based on the current management and leadership styles, or external ones dependent on the effects from outside competition

Strengths, Weaknesses, Opportunities, and Threats (SWOT) Analysis: A structured form of analysis to better understand the current positioning of an individual or company in its appropriate competitive landscape

Applications

Eye care practices do not work in a vacuum. The usual situation includes other practices, both private and academic, that compete for the same patient. All the different businesses that provide the same services (eg, diabetic retinal screening) or products (eg, glasses from optical) combine to define the competitive landscape. Exceling in this environment requires the ability to effectively differentiate and appropriately position your practice. This then draws patients to you.

The challenge is that the practice's internal and external environments are in a state of constant change. There is a continuous competition both inside and outside the company that influences the climate. Employees are trying to earn raises and move up the organizational ladder, and competitors are working to drive patients toward themselves.

Effective leaders acknowledge this dynamic environment and embrace the need for change. This process requires 2 steps. The first is to understand what is going on for a particular issue in the competitive landscape and how the practice is positioned for it. There are many tools that help in this assessment. One example is a SWOT Analysis (Figure 1-1). This form helps identify the critical factors influencing the current condition. The analysis breaks the problem down to strengths, weaknesses, opportunities, and threats. It forces the user to view the issue with different lenses, or viewpoints, to get a complete sense of the environment. This facilitates the development of ideas and strategies to address the needs.

The second step to initiating change is actually doing it in the practice. Unlike step 1 that involves a business-only approach that is void of feelings, step 2 requires skills to deal with the more complex nature of people. Great leadership understands that change is typically defied but uses effective strategies to overcome it. This is where having the right culture, as demonstrated by leaders, pays dividends.

Leaders use a 2-pronged approach by explaining the need for the change and then addressing the dread of change by offering sympathy. Remember, treat the staff like adults and expect them to behave that way. This includes a statement like, "The conversion from paper to electronic records is required for us to continue practicing

Figure 1-1. Example of a SWOT Analysis.

SWOT Analysis			
Issue: Converting Paper to Electronic Records			
Strengths	Weaknesses	Opportunities	Threats
*IT staff in-house *Capable staff with IT experience	*Lack of hardware and software *Lack of compatibility with diagnostics	*Earn extra payment from incentives *Streamline operations with eRx and eReferrals	*Eventual penalty if not implemented *Perpetual inefficiencies with drug prescribing

and avoid penalties." It is then followed up with a comment to sympathize but also motive the team such as, "I understand and feel the same anxiety about this change. Therefore, technical support will be available to help in anticipation of any challenges you may encounter. I know we can find a way to be even better as a team after this obstacle." If leadership has created the right culture and follows through by modeling the correct behavior, followers will join the ride.

Immediate Action Items

Identify 2 or 3 important issues facing your practice not only today, but also in the future. Common questions involve the adoption of electronic medical records, diversification of payer mix, and company expansion through locations and additional doctors. Practice creating a SWOT analysis for each of these problems. However, do not let this overwhelm you because almost certainly you will realize you do not have all the answers or know all the information. That is ok. This is a tool to get our juices flowing and help direct you to specific questions where more information is needed. It is in this process that you will arrive at one of the most important realizations when leading change or facing any other problem—you recognize what you do not know. This is the first real step, self-assessment, that will orient you down the right path. Without it, you do not even realize that you do not know there is a problem. The more you practice this process, the easier it will become. You will soon develop better solutions in shorter time periods, which leads to superior outcomes. Other chapters later in this book will help fill in some of those missing pieces you encountered in this process.

Developing the Talent

Importance

Although the most desirable businesses can more easily draw in gifted individuals from outside of their organization, they also look within their own staff to identity and develop talent that might be special. This enables a business to tap into a diverse set of skillful employees, both externally and internally. The result is a steady filling of open positions with the best people that fit the company's needs.

For this to occur in your practice, the leadership team must provide the opportunity and possess the required abilities to train those unpolished individuals. One admirable trait that is highlighted with this behavior is that those in charge of training are willing to teach others the same skills that would make the trainers obsolete. The psychological undertone is that those individuals are secure enough in themselves to share these lessons.[1] Outstanding leaders realize the importance of having great leadership in their own businesses. They consider it a priority to teach about leadership even if this means they are mentoring those that may replace or compete with them in the future. These individuals place the success of the organization before their own. This altruistic culture they create and propagate supports the principles stated in the practice's vision and mission statements.

Keywords

Job enlargement: An action taken to increase the task load for an employee

Development: A process of improvement through learning, experiencing, and maturing

Mentorship: A process where an experienced individual passes along knowledge and provides guidance with the goal of developing another person

Human nature: The innate qualities and behaviors of a human being

Character: The summation of a person's values, beliefs, and attributes

Applications

Practices always benefit from having great talent among their staff. We never come across businesses that feel they would be better off with employees that are not good. The trouble is this pool of sought-after talent is both limited and expensive. The more common situation a practice faces is trying to juggle having the best employees but at the right price. One method to address this challenge is to develop individuals from within the company. This is possible because not all new employees that are hired will be refined. In certain positions, like work-up technicians, the turnover is so high that new hires routinely need to be trained.

Effective job enlargement can be a tremendous asset to a practice. This requires having a process in place that permits the growth and identifies the right individuals. Leaders understand and appreciate the value of having talented individuals around them. Therefore, they are the ideal candidates to provide the mentorship needed for the employee development. Leaders also understand human nature. They can connect and encourage those they are mentoring for job enlargement while modeling the behavior needed to exemplify it.[3]

The other part of this challenge is to find employees with the right character and competency to blossom with the training. This is an instance of when having good Human Resources will help find those diamonds in the rough. Appropriate employee evaluation and performance review isolates those employees that have the desire to grow along with the necessary skill set and values to flourish. The practical application would be to connect a rookie technician to a Certified Ophthalmic Assistant (COA), a COA to a Certified Ophthalmic Technician (COT), and then a COT to the Director of Operations. This creates a culture where growth is encouraged and expected as well. It also demonstrates a sense of priority to have every employee be a vital member of the whole team.

Immediate Action Items

Does your practice have a system in place, such as annual performance reviews, where employees are asked about their short- and long-term professional goals? This would include achievements that may or may not be reachable in your organization. If so, develop some plan where suitable leaders that have experience related to those aspirations can mentor the employee. Remember that the ability to provide mentorship is also a skill set that needs to be learned and similarly needs to be trained in those that will mentor. It is a continual process with everyone learning and then passing down that knowledge to others. This works best when a culture is in place that fosters and encourages the desired behavior.

If not, then dedicate a portion of time to ask thought-provoking questions to your employees about what they really want to do in their lives. Allow them to discuss options that may not be possible or related to their current position in your organization. Realize that, as great leaders, your responsibility is to allow those with special talent and desires to spread their wings and fly, as opposed to caging them into a confined space. Even if this individual eventually leaves the organization to pursue other goals, your current employees will see and respect the developmental process that occurred. This will excite them to actively take part in their own growth process.

Empowering the Employees

Importance

There is a common misconception about the relationship between those that lead vs those that follow. It is thought that demonstrating great leadership requires a leader that is the best at, and does, everything. To the contrary, this situation is usually an example of an inefficient use of resources.

Although a leader may be able to do all the functions required in a given settings, great leadership does not typically exhibit that behavior. Instead, excellent leaders use their valuable knowledge to take a different approach. First, they have a firm understanding of their followers' strengths and weaknesses. Second, they are aware of what the company needs in a given situation. They then know where and how to position these human resources to achieve the optimal response.

Great leaders know the people around them. The information they gather does not just happen by accident. They understand and value each individual relationship with their followers. In an ideal setting, there would be infinite time to focus on these interactions. However, the real world presents challenges that limit these opportunities to build quality relationships. The best leaders maximize the time they do have with each person. They use the information gained from the bonding experiences to get the most out of the employees when needed. The result is a culture that benefits from all the available talent to create an environment of sustainable efficiency and successful outcomes.

Keywords

Job enrichment: The process of enabling job enlargement for an employee along with the addition of autonomy to perform those required tasks

Empowerment: The act of giving support and providing autonomy to an individual or group that allows them to make and follow through on their own decisions

Vertical leadership: A leadership structure where leaders are positioned at the top of a hierarchical-based organization with the authority to give direction while those at the bottom follow orders and provide information upward

Horizontal leadership: A leadership structure where direction is given and information is shared in a side-to-side direction as authority is more spread out over the organization

Applications

Job enlargement, which elevates employees higher in the organization structure, is not the only way to maximize talent. Another avenue for opportunity is developing staff to broaden their current position through job enrichment. This improves productivity by giving employees more responsibility by additional autonomy to accomplish their goals. The underlying principle is the use of empowerment.

Great leaders understand that they do not and should not be doing all the work in a group setting. In fact, the leader may not even be the best skilled to perform a given task. True leadership values the qualities of every individual. Their role is to position each member in the right spot to optimize their skills to accomplish a given task.[7] They provide the necessary resources to be successful and allow individuals to demonstrate their unique talents by taking on responsibility. Effective leaders allow their followers to make mistakes and use them as opportunities to evaluate and improve individuals.

An example of this is having the Director of Operations give a senior COT the responsibility to create and maintain the work schedule for all the other technicians. This mentorship from the Director to the COT transfers a task under the responsibility of the Director to that of the COT. The Director provides the necessary templates and ground rules along with the autonomy to take over. Once the COT has had the opportunity to perform this task, the Director circles back to provide evaluation and constructive feedback. This process allows for and encourages continued improvement while strengthening the working relationship between the two. The result is horizontal growth through job enrichment and leaves the whole practice better off by maximizing resources.

The best situation is a combination of job enrichment and job enlargement. It enables both vertical and horizontal leadership. This improves the practice by utilizing inherent efficiencies and developing more talented staff. It also models a winning culture.

Immediate Action Items

Do you routinely ask yourself, along with other high-ranking employees, if some of the tasks you perform can be delegated to someone further down the organizational chart? In other words, is your time being used to complete activities that only you are skilled and qualified to accomplish? If so, continue to pass along the nonessential tasks. This will help identify those with special talents and desires as it will provide them an opportunity to grow and demonstrate their skill set. Remember that, although others can be capable of performing these activities, this does not mean that they are trained and ready to execute them. You must have a system in place that allows for the individual to obtain the necessary knowledge and opportunity to practice the function. Allow them to make mistakes. Create a positive environment where development is encouraged, and not one of anxiety where mistakes are reprimanded.

However, if you are not doing this delegation, then your organization is working inefficiently. Not only is the high-priced human resource, such as yourself, performing duties that do not provide the best return on the invested time, but also the lower-priced employees are not being optimized and likely have unoccupied, or idle time, on their hands. Identify and pass along nonessential functions to those that have the capability to execute them. This will achieve 2 goals. First, it improves the company's financial status. Second, it creates a positive work environment and culture that demonstrates individuals higher in the organization chart trust to delegate responsibility downward to responsive employees.

Encouraging Teamwork

Importance

In any organization, individuals are placed in positions where they need to work in teams to complete tasks. The accepted belief in these situations is that the whole is greater than the sum of its parts. The ability to achieve this synergy among different individuals is easier said than done. The intrinsic differences among people requires either an individual to lead the activity with an emphasis on teamwork or have an organizational process in place that expects the correct behavior.

Extraordinary businesses have leadership that understands and promote the use of teamwork in their organization. The goal is to achieve a company dynamic where uniquely skilled employees can come together to evaluate problems, develop answers, and execute actions. This ability to construct team-oriented, problem-solving groups allows companies to remain productive in a dynamically competitive environment. It does this by maximizing the human resources by valuing diversity.

Keywords

Self-directed work team: A group of individuals that by themselves have the ability to identify, assess, plan, and execute actions when faced with problems

Diversity: A quality of having a mixture of backgrounds, values, and beliefs that can help provide advantages that could not be achieved with a more homogenous set of individuals

Brainstorm: The process of discussing issues and allowing the individuals of the group to generate possible solutions

Motivation: The act of providing encouragement to another person to achieve a goal

Employee investment: The belief that when employees are given the opportunity to take part in the steps of addressing a problem that they will be motivated to see its success

Applications

The natural diversity that arises from a group of individuals represents an opportunity to create value. Leaders cherish these differences. It provides them a wide range of resources that they can combine to create a solution that addresses every unique problem. A basic example is the extraordinary customer service a practice can offer to an ethnically varied patient population by having technicians that speak different languages.

Great leadership unites a heterogeneous employee base to function as a group. The challenge is developing a team approach where it is both valued and expected that individuals help one another for the benefit of the group. The best teams are ones that can anticipate, recognize, strategize, and react to problems in the workplace. These self-directed work teams are empowered by their leaders to effectively brainstorm ideas that capitalize on their diversity to strategically create solutions. This process not only optimizes company resources but also gives the employees a sense of value and trust, which can be priceless. Motivation and employee investment drive the team to create a successful result when they are given the autonomy to make decisions. They have skin in the game because their credibility is on the line.

An example of such a powerful team is when the Director of Operations challenges a group of front office staff and technicians to improve patient flow through the clinic. This collection of different individuals and roles look for cases when flow is inefficient, brainstorm ideas, and generate solutions to be implemented. The Director reviews the proposed plan, provides feedback, and executes the plan with the team. The process reinforces the targeted culture of encouraging teamwork and valuing diversity in the practice.

Immediate Action Items

Does your practice encourage the utilization of teams to address complex issues? If so, this is a great start. Are the team members static or do they change in a dynamic manner? Consider every individual in an organization to have a unique set of qualities, just like every piece in a jigsaw puzzle. The key to success is valuing what each brings to the team. In the process of problem solving, make sure to ask and observe what everyone's skill set is. Incorporate this information to mix and match the composite abilities of the practice to methodically address challenges.

If you do not use teams, then it is time to incorporate the philosophy that better results occur from a group of individuals complementing one another vs what any one of them could accomplish by themselves. Identify a small yet unaddressed problem in your practice that, if solved, would result in a benefit for the organization. Create a functional and diverse team of staff members based on knowledge from your leadership team, then present them with the problem and offer resources both to arrive at and execute their plan of action. Practice this model many times with increasing difficulty in the problem. Naturally, this will allow for more complex issues to be addressed. The key is for the leader governing this activity to recognize 2 things. First, allow your team to do their job and hold them accountable to it. Second, it is the job of the leader to provide the team with the necessary environment and tools needed for them to be successful. Everyone is responsible for the outcome of the project.

Managing Conflict

Importance

One uncontested truth in life is that anytime there are 2 or more individuals interacting together, there will be a disagreement at some point about a topic. This is a natural consequence because no 2 people think exactly the same way on all issues. The important takeaway is to anticipate that conflict will inevitably occur. Although the goal in an organization is to implement strategies and create a culture that thrives on differences, the successful leader understands how to effectively deal with problems that may arise.

The benefits of conflict management appear to only involve those of the initial parties at first glance; however, effective resolution counseling provides many benefits that are felt throughout the organization. It allows employees a method to convert a situation that can cause feelings of anger and resentment into a productive activity where various viewpoints are encouraged, which lead to unified solutions. The downstream effect is the development and maintenance of a company culture that promotes teamwork for the benefit of the entire organization. This also eliminates the discussion and involvement of Human Resources should the disagreement take a negative course.

Keywords

Conflict resolution: The process of identifying and addressing problems between individuals

Conflict of interest: The condition that exists when the actions of one individual might be affected by outside influences that provide benefit to the individual for a particular behavior

Attributes: The qualities or traits of a person

Applications

Leadership will always be tested with conflict resolution in a company because staff will naturally disagree. The value of great leaders is evident as the results of these confrontations can vary significantly. Effectively managing conflict reverts back to the successful implementation of the right culture. The first challenge is to remove any emotions that can play a role and focus only on objective facts. This reduces conflicts of interest. If the culture is set for everyone to behave professionally, this can occur devoid of feelings. Employees that resist performing to these expectations should be noted to Human Resources for inclusion into their review.

The next step is to bring the conflicting sides together and reframe the situation. Instead of pitting one against the other, the best leaders unite the 2 together under a common theme. This promotes teamwork and not opposition. Most individuals have good human nature and mean to do well. It should not be surprising that a vast majority of these conflicts occur because of a lack of communication between 2 well-intentioned individuals.

Consider an eye care provider who increasingly notices that his glaucoma patients presenting for their clinical visits are not having a visual field performed right before they are seen by him. He tells the Director of Operations to fix the problem. The Director first tries to get the objective facts from each side. The scribe working with the doctor expresses her frustration that the front office staff is not scheduling correctly. She always writes the order on the exit sheet used with the patient's prior encounter. The problem is brought to the front office employee. He appears tired of hearing these complaints of his inability to schedule correctly. He is following the instructions on how to do it given by his supervisor and believes there must not have been an order for a visual field.

Good leadership notices this brewing hostility. The Director brings them together to reach a solution. Without letting emotions manipulate the conversation, the leader orients the discussion toward teamwork and problem solving. The following would be an effective approach:

> Beth and Tony, I am glad we could meet to talk. I understand clinic can get very busy, and I see that both of you are working hard. Thank you for your efforts. Dr. Teymoorian has challenged us to fix the problem with his visual field scheduling. I had a chance to discuss this with both of you. Each of you is doing the right thing. This turns out to be an operational and communication issue. Beth is marking down the need for a visual field at the top of the exit form while Tony has been trained to look at the bottom. In the future, if you are notice any similar issues, I encourage you to bring them up so we can proactively address the problem as a team. Our organization values your experience and commitment. We encourage and expect this high level of thoughtfulness to our processes. Again, thank you.

Immediate Action Items

Does your organization have formalized training for the leadership team on how to manage conflict and arrive at resolutions? If so, are there processes in place that coordinate the results of these activities with the employees' human resource records? It is important that if time is spent to manage conflicts among staff members that any corrective action be noted in the respective files. This documentation becomes valuable at times of annual reviews, which can eventually lead to many results, anywhere from promotion to termination. Without written evidence, any Human Resources actions taken by the company exposes it to legal risk and usually wasted money along with time. If not, then collaborate with Human Resources to make sure these activities are properly documented.

For those practices that do not have training in place, many resources exist that provide it with strategies and steps on how to approach conflict management. Allocate time for your leadership team to be educated in these methods, which include taking part in fake scenarios to practice these skills. It is already difficult enough trying to mediate in real situations as emotions can run high. Therefore, preparations on how to handle these issues must be done ahead of time to be effective.

CRITICAL LEADERSHIP POINTERS

* Culture is an organization's compass; every employee and process reverts back to it for guidance on how to behave and what is expected.
* Leaders must always exemplify the culture they wish to have in an organization because people are always watching.
* It is important to both know what good leadership is and how it is modeled.
* The role of a leader is not the same as a manager in a business.
* A great leader knows how to follow and does follow at times.
* An individual does not need to have the highest position to lead because anyone can lead from any position in an organization.
* First, learn everyone's name in your organization; and second, get to know something important about them so you build a strong connection.
* Although an increase in pay is always welcomed, employees deep down appreciate when leaders acknowledge the value and importance of their work; do not forget to thank people.
* Diversity creates some of the most valuable assets for a leader, especially when they have a team composed of players placed in the right positions with a complementary culture that encourages collaborative behavior.
* Diversity creates some of the most difficult challenges for a leader, especially when they must deal with a conflict within a culture that values the individual over the team.

REFERENCES

1. Maxwell JC. *The 21 Irrefutable Laws of Leadership*. Nashville, TN: Thomas Nelson, Incorporated; 2007.
2. Kouzes JM, Posner BZ. *The Truth About Leadership*. San Francisco, CA: Jossey-Bass; 2010.
3. Maxwell JC. *Becoming a Person of Influence*. Nashville, TN: Thomas Nelson, Incorporated; 1997.
4. Ittelson TR. *Financial Statements*. Pompton Plains, NJ: Career Press; 2009.
5. Kotter JP. *Leading Change*. Boston, MA: Harvard Business Review Press; 1996.
6. Kamauff J. *Manager's Guide to Operations Management*. Madison, WI: The McGraw-Hill Companies, Incorporated.
7. Maxwell JC. *Developing the Leader Within You*. Nashville, TN: Thomas Nelson, Incorporated; 1993.

2

Understanding Organizational Behavior

Growing a culture requires a good storyteller.
Changing a culture requires a persuasive editor.

— Ryan Lilly

INTRODUCTION

Although understanding an organization's vision is important, a clear architectural plan laying out a company's structure and inner dynamics is essential. It provides the fundamental rules and regulations that govern the employees' work and their interactions among themselves. An effective leadership team in an eye care practice utilizes this framework to foster a winning culture. It recognizes the value created by this interplay and capitalizes on it to differentiate the company in the competitive marketplace.

Organizational behavior (OB) is the study of how individuals interact with each other and as a group. It focuses on the framework and social order in a business. Common examples of OB include the reporting order of how a technician seeks supervision, the way an employee treats other staff members and patients, and the directional flow of information from higher-level supervisors like the Chief Executive Officer to lower-level staff.

Practitioners are typically either at or near the apex in the hierarchical structure within an organization. Consequently, they are accountable for exemplifying and supporting the targeted culture. Their ability to perform this duty dramatically impacts the company as it demonstrates the expected employee conduct. The result

Teymoorian S. *Essential Business Fundamentals for the Successful Eye Care Practice* (pp 21-37).
© 2019 SLACK Incorporated.

is that the everyday actions of the providers influence and shape the company's behavioral pattern.

This chapter addresses the fundamentals about organizational design and the functions within it. First, it starts with a discussion about how businesses are organized in terms of their mechanical structure and cultural philosophy. Attention then turns to the different types of supervisory and subordinate styles. These core topics then build up to an examination about company dynamics. The objective of this chapter involves enabling the eye care practitioner to successfully take the vision established from leadership and convert it to the application of a strategy in an organization.

What Is Organizational Behavior?

All businesses have 2 fundamental characteristics. Both of these center on the fact that human beings are essential for some, if not all, of their processes. The first is the need for structured reporting among the individuals. The second is the influence of these interactions on the company culture.[1] On the surface, it may appear that these findings are not critical. The reality is that the interaction between individuals and the organization has repercussions that resonate throughout the entire business.

Nonetheless, these topics can be neglected easily in organizations despite their importance. This can especially occur in smaller companies because the bulk of the limited attention goes to profit-generating activities. However, businesses that thrive for extended periods of time have unambiguous messaging about their structure and culture. This does not imply that the structure needs to be rigid and the culture formal. There are many successful organizations that have other identities. The key is to align the company goals with a structure and culture that supports it. This assumes the business has good leadership and thoughtful objectives as discussed earlier in this book. Employees are then left with a clear understanding of what is expected from them and how they should behave.

Once the structure and culture are understood, they need to be demonstrated by the individuals in the organization. This task is not as simple as telling the employees to act a certain way. The complexity arises because we are dealing with humans—no 2 are the same. This requires appreciating their uniqueness and comprehending the different ways individuals react in certain roles and conditions. Companies are inherently left to proceed in either of 2 pathways as a result. The easier option is to ignore these variations and take whatever result occurs. This is like trying to pass only round pegs into a hole with the hope they will be the right size and shape. The result is a company made of only round pegs of a certain size. The other choice is to test both round and triangular pegs through the opening. The latter method utilizes all that is available by being accepting of diversity. The flourishing practitioner understands that both a round and triangular peg are valuable assets to possess.

ORGANIZATIONAL BEHAVIOR IN EYE CARE

The relevance of studying OB in eye care is to enable the maximization of the company's most important and expensive resource: its employees. The application of OB affects everyone because individuals in a company do not work in a vacuum. The resulting interaction, however, can be quite complex. The way they engage with one another has a significant impact on the organization's culture. Also, the associated reporting lines directly influence the day-to-day operations. Top organizations understand the importance of this dependence among its employees. They give time and effort to nurture and orient these relationships. The necessary skills in OB for the successful provider to demonstrate are incorporating organizational structure, optimizing organizational culture, comprehending supervisory philosophies, appreciating subordinate styles, and navigating company dynamics.

Incorporating Organizational Structure

Importance

People mistakenly believe that a formal internal structure is needed only for large corporations with many employees. However, all entities from professional organizations, such as companies, to social groups, such as families, benefit from order for its members. An organized structure with transparent reporting patterns provides the basic framework in a business for its operations. It defines every member's role and relationship relative to others. This eliminates awkward and possibly hurtful interpersonal situations that can occur both with and without intention. Prosperous companies strategically implement a logical framework to optimize their employees' production and facilitate a healthy work environment. The effect is a successful business that maintains a positive culture.

The ability to accomplish this feat has far-reaching, beneficial influence throughout the entire organization. The most obvious areas are those in operations and Human Resources. Unambiguous reporting lines provide employees a guideline for conduct. Clear expectations encourage accountability among staff and subsequently decrease conflicts that need to involve intervention from Human Resources.. Once employees are held responsible for their actions, they have personal ownership to the outcomes of their decisions, whether good or bad. This accountability, for most individuals, improves their performance because the results of these choices reflect back on the employees themselves. This dramatically improves operational processes and outcomes.

If there are any changes in reporting duties, such as those seen with organizational restructuring, it is imperative to update the staff right away with a revised chart. Situations that leave employees without order commonly result in many more problems, both professionally and socially. The shock of restructuring can be uncomfortable by itself. The addition of new, undefined relationships magnifies the issues.

Keywords

Organizational behavior (OB): The study of how individuals and groups behave and interact with another in an organization

Organizational framework: The manner in which a company is organized into its structure

Organizational chart: A diagram where reporting lines are used to illustrate the roles of each individual and their relationship to one another

Formalization: The degree in which an organization is run by official rules of conduct and behavior

Socialization: The way an organization is run by social rules of conduct and behavior

Direct report: A type of reporting in an organization where one individual is immediately in charge of another one

Indirect report: A type of reporting in an organization where layers of intermediate reporting exist between individuals

Solid line: A type of line used in organizational charts denoting authority from a supervisor to a subordinate

Dashed line: A type of line used in organizational charts denoting functional authority to give tasks to others, but not as a direct supervisor

Dotted line: A type of line used in organizational charts denoting authority to only give advice to an individual

Applications

Employees rely on the leadership team to provide them with structure.[1] This framework is important because it imparts a sense of boundary, order, and relationship in the organization. The manner in which the workers interact with one another shapes the organizational culture. Each practice should take on its own unique structural framework that optimizes the behavior of its staff.

The most important application from OB is the creation and use of an organizational chart. This chart carefully delineates the relationship among all the members of the practice and removes confusion. It helps each individual employee understand from whom to take direction and to whom to answer, which may not be the same individual. The formalization of the chart depends on the degree of the company's culture to follow official rules. This is opposite from the amount of socialization where social rules and construct define its culture.

Consider this example of an organizational chart from Teymoorian Eye Associates. It focuses on Beth, a front office staff employee (Figure 2-1). The diagram visually explains the relationship she has with every other staff member. This scheme also dictates the interaction type between the connected employees. She is a direct report of the Front Office Manager, and an indirect report of the Director of Operations and the Physician Owner. The solid line means that Beth's immediate boss is Front Office Manager. She provides Beth the majority of her supervisory duties. The dashed lines to the Technician Manager and the Director of Finance represent that they can give direct orders for Beth to follow; however, Beth still reports to the Front Office

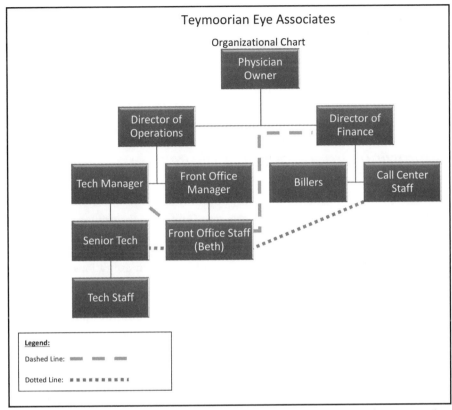

Figure 2-1. Example of an organizational chart demonstrating the different types of reporting orders.

Manager. The dotted lines indicate that Beth and the Senior Technicians along with the Call Center Staff collaborate, but they do not give orders to Beth.

Immediate Action Items

Does your practice have a formalized organization chart? If so, is it updated and does every staff member either know it or where to look it up? If it is current, that is wonderful news. The key is to keep it that way when there are any new changes. If not, then carefully assess the present chart and critically evaluate how the new chart should look. It is very important to develop a correct one because it will be tested and critiqued by the entire organization. To avoid unexpected negative reactions, attempt to consider as many different viewpoints as possible. Reporting lines and how they are drawn can easily unveil contentious office politics and their associated drama due in part to the formalization of being written down. However, this should not prevent a chart from being made because any successful company needs clear structure.

If you do not have a chart, then it is time to create one. However, do not rush and present a chart to your staff without first thinking it out carefully. Once it is shown to the staff, you will need to be ready to answer questions on how it works but also be open to uncomfortable discussions if some members are not happy. First, develop a chart that illustrates how the company is currently run. Second, thoughtfully contemplate and create one based on where you want the practice to be as defined by the vision and mission statement. Third, provide a chart that can help bridge the current to the future version based on what is possible at the current moment given the available human resources. Then, as the company develops over time, utilize the information from the future chart to make the correct personnel and associated work relationship changes to get to the desired state.

Optimizing Organizational Culture

Importance

The best companies realize the importance of culture as the driving force leading their employees. The challenge persists to continually align the organization's culture with its goals. Employees naturally behave in a manner that attempts to achieve the company objectives when they are aligned with their own aspirations. Otherwise, their actions create outcomes that are not prioritized by the organization. This results in wasted resources and frustrated staff.

Elite practices promote the ideal culture and provide the environmental support to continually propagate it. However, the employees are the ones creating and using it. One unexpected feature of culture is that any individual can play the role of leader and follower. In a business with an undefined culture, the leaders demonstrate culture to the followers. These followers are now armed with an understanding of it. If properly empowered, they will teach those unfamiliar with it. This cycle continues throughout the organization and even can loop back to those initially involved in the process.

One vital challenge that high-level organizations pass is sustaining the favored culture over time. Similar to a game of telephone, the message that is sent from one individual to the next can change subtly depending on how it is heard, interpreted, and passed along through the process. This is where strong leadership intervenes at different times throughout the spreading of information to ensure the message stays on point. What this means is that leaders must continually model the right behavior. Successful completion of this task produces a strong and time-tested culture that permeates throughout the entire company.

Keywords

Downward communication: An organizational communication style where information is transferred from the top of a hierarchy to the bottom

Upward communication: An organizational communication style where information is transferred from the bottom of a hierarchy to the top

Lateral communication: An organizational communication style where information is transferred side-to-side in a hierarchy

Champion: An employee or customer that strongly believes in and promotes a company

Applications

Elite practices utilize different approaches to reach the targeted culture. Leaders are the influential forces that either create a new culture or reshape a previously existing one. However, the process of having a positive culture goes beyond the first few steps initiated by a leader. The challenge is to strengthen and spread it throughout the organization to reach the masses. The recruitment of followers is required to pass along the message. This is another example of the value gained through empowerment. Every employee has a unique skill set and can make a significant contribution to the team when given the proper opportunity and support.

Strategic leaders are always looking out for situations to convert their trained and resourceful followers into exemplary leaders. The difficulty is providing the right environment to allow the followers to relay the message. The best practices catalyze this reaction by creating conditions where individuals can lead and demonstrate the culture from any position in the organization. This relies heavily on the ability to create meaningful communication pathways that link the individual employees together.

Communication is a vehicle to express culture. Average businesses follow a strict tradition of downward communication. This scenario only permits information to be transferred down. It limits the opportunity to demonstrate leadership to only those at the top. This flawed behavior assumes that only those superior employees have ability and vision, and everyone else is simply a tool to be used in the process. However, thriving practices recognize every employee's value. They encourage communication in all directions, including downward along with upward and lateral.

Consider Richard, the Technician Manager at Teymoorian Eye Associates (Figure 2-2). His central position in the organization chart permits him direct contact with much of the staff. He is hardworking and supports the goals of the practice. Some would even consider him a champion for the company. Nonetheless, he does not want to step on anyone's toes. His concern for not creating any trouble is enough that he even limits his champion behavior to not draw attention to himself.

The practice can easily overlook the opportunity to have Richard lead from within the organization. The result is that those around him will not benefit from his exemplary behavior and attitude. Average companies either do not see his value or do not have the right environment in place to capitalize on it. A better approach is to have an established culture where his contributions are treasured. The Director of Operations should recognize and empower Richard to express his beliefs. This will happen if the Director was trained by the Physician Owner to behave the same way.

Immediate Action Items

Do your staff members have safe and open communication methods with the leadership team for both their satisfactions and concerns? Take a survey of some employees and ask them, "Do you feel comfortable to raise your thoughts about our practice?" Anything less than a convincing answer along with how it would be done leaves space for improvement. If this is the case, then chances are the current company culture does not match its favored state. Incorporate the leadership strategies in this book to first identify the ideal culture and make sure to align it with

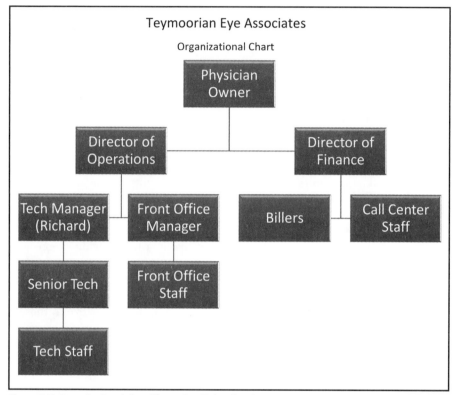

Figure 2-2. Organizational chart illustrating Richard's role.

complementing vision and mission statements. Then, apply the information from the rest of the text to model and enhance the culture. Each of these areas will, in one form or another, contribute the success or downfall of the culture.

Comprehending Supervisory Philosophies

Importance

By nature, the presence of organizational structure creates supervisor and subordinate positions. The interactions between these groups shape the business and play a significant role in the success of the company. The best businesses appreciate the variability in each of these positions and use that diversity to achieve goals.[1]

The important point to remember is that the way supervisors govern needs to complement the organizational culture and align with its goals. This does not mean that each supervisor within one company needs to use a particular style all the time. The ideal situation is one where supervisors remain flexible in the fluid workplace. The reality is static companies generally do not last over a long period of time. They are either unwilling or unable to adapt to its internal environment and external landscape. As subordinates and competitors change, great supervisors assess the situation and make changes that ensure that resources are used efficiently and outcomes are maximized.

One particular note is that this does not imply that supervisors must alter their style in every new setting. Sometimes it is best to remain consistent with methods if anticipated changes are counterproductive to the desired culture and goals. This stresses the importance of having strong leadership in place to reinforce the actions needed to continually support the company's vision and mission.

Keywords

Personal construct: The way in which an individual sees, interprets, and interacts with the world

Stereotype: The attribution of certain qualities to another person based on their group membership, such as gender or race

Expertise: The quality of having experience in an area or field

Power: The degree to which an individual can exude control over others

Directive style: A fast thought process that bases decisions on information in order to proceed to the next topic

Task-oriented behavior: A style of decision making that focuses on getting objectives met

Behavioral style: A slow thought process that bases decisions on how it will influence others

Relationship-oriented behavior: A style of decision making that focuses on relationship building

Conceptual style: A thought process that bases decisions on its effect on larger-scale themes

Applications

The quality of employee interaction in a practice is a major influence for its well-being. This includes how supervisors and their subordinates behave with one another. It would be easy to have a cookie-cutter approach to guide these relationships, but human beings are complex; all have their own personal constructs and stereotypes. What works in a particular setting may not translate to the next one. The top practices accept these differences. They create an overall philosophy of what should occur and then allow the employees to work together to figure things out. This approach maintains structure but allows for individuality.

Employees in supervisory roles are expected to possess a level of expertise. This instills power in their positions. The way that power is utilized can vary significantly and determines the supervisor's effectiveness. The hope is that the established organizational culture guides these managers to use their power in a productive manner.[1] This example reiterates the importance of maintaining the ideal culture in a practice.

Three general supervisory styles exist and each can be incorporated to meet the needs of the practice. Supervisors that use a directive style will obtain as much information as possible and then make a decision. This style coincides with task-oriented behavior that strives to get tasks completed. Subordinates working in this environment will be asked to help gather the needed data in an accurate and efficient manner. The goal is completing line items on an agenda.

Behavioral style is another approach to supervision. This style places value on how decisions affect the relationships on those involved in making them. This serves a relationship-oriented behavior where the goal of the decision-making process is to create valued bonds among people. This then translates into the process of gathering information to make choices. It is a slower pace than the directive style because team-building generally takes more time than data collection.

The third method of supervision is a conceptual style. This method attempts to make choices based on the effect to larger-scaled themes. The thought process involves analyzing how each decision will influence greater concepts, such as culture. Its characteristics will be determined by the theme with which it tries to align.

The strategic advantage to these various approaches is to acknowledge that differences exist and understand how the supervisor goes about getting work done. Although all methods can be functional, diversity in these methods helps add value to the practice. The next step is to link these styles with those of the subordinates.

Immediate Action Items

What is your type of supervisory style: directive, behavioral, or conceptual? Most individuals tend to follow one more than any other. Take a moment to appreciate the other types that do exist. Now list a few problems that currently exist in your organization. Would applying a different style create some opportunities or even solutions to these issues? This approach can uncover subtle findings or viewpoints you had never considered. You may be surprised to see that your interaction with subordinates improves as your new style better fits their philosophy. If this new dynamic aligns with favored culture, it is ok to incorporate this method to better maximize the working relationship. However, if it does not, then utilizing it will model behavior that undermines the company's goals.

Appreciating Subordinate Styles

Importance

The behavioral styles of subordinates provide as much variety as the supervisors that manage them. Effective organizations realize that one major task of their supervisors is the need to handle these differences to get the most from their subordinates' production. They should be given the necessary tools and resources to deal with these variations. This demonstrates another example of how such challenges are viewed differently in great vs average companies. Exemplary businesses accept this as an opportunity to permit employee growth and empowerment while ordinary ones deal with it as a burden. This circles back to the organizational culture and the quality of leadership in place.

Similarly to supervisors, this situation does not imply that subordinate behavioral styles should remain the same over time. Successful organizations hire quality employees through their Human Resources that have the ability to change in a manner that best fits the needs of the company. The burden of this responsibility is divided between the supervisor and the subordinate. The supervisor should remain flexible to the style of the subordinate. At the same time, the supervisor must be able to request and initiate change in the subordinate when that action is warranted.

This situation illustrates 2 critical points in the hiring process. The first is the need for Human Resources to properly hire talent. It includes individuals that possess these adaptable abilities to change and the commitment to help the organization reach its goals. The second is the importance for leadership to provide Human Resources a clear message about the company's vision and mission.

Keywords

Affective commitment: An employee's decision to remain with a company based on emotional connection

Normative commitment: An employee's decision to remain with a company based on a feeling of obligation

Continuance commitment: An employee's decision to remain with a company based on the degree of difficulties that would arise from changing employment

Equity theory: A method of employee thinking that uses the treatment of others as a reference point on how appropriately the individual is being treated in an organization

Reinforcement theory: A method of employee thinking that alters the employees behavioral actions based on perceived consequences

Positive reinforcement: The use of giving beneficial rewards to employees who demonstrate the desired behavior in an organization

Negative reinforcement: The use of giving penalties to employees who do not demonstrate the desired behavior in an organization

Turnover: The percentage of employees that depart and are replaced relative to the number of total employees in an organization

Skill-based pay method: A merit-based system that rewards employees that grow their skill set and meet certain milestones in development

Burnout: An extreme condition in which employees have exhausted their ability to properly work anymore

Wellness program: A support system within an organization that focuses on employee well-being, including the issue of burnout

Applications

One factor to consider, before analyzing subordinate behavioral patterns, is to recognize the different reasons why subordinates stay at a practice. There are a few to consider. Those with an affective commitment have an emotional tie with the company. This connection can stem from their job satisfaction such as taking care of people's eyes. The individuals with a normative commitment remain at the practice due to a sense of obligation. This feeling can be toward other staff members or to the company itself. These employees do not want to break an agreement because they value the principle of keeping promises. Another type is the continuance commitment. This centers around the belief that the sacrifices required to make a transition to another company is not worth its reward. Examples of these losses range from leaving friendships with other employees to forfeiting job security. A critical note to realize is that, regardless of the commitment type, a positive culture that values its employees and provides meaningful work will always be difficult to leave to go elsewhere. The information learned about employees' commitment types becomes valuable as a forecasting tool on what behavior to expect in other situations. This supplies their supervisors an understanding of how to approach them to maximize their efforts.

There are 2 prevailing concepts about how subordinates perceive work. These complement the prior discussion about commitment. The equity theory views interactions and the decision-making process as one of equality or fairness. These employees are satisfied as long as they perceive similar treatment to those in comparable positions. The benefit is that actions can be justified on the basis on keeping equality. The downside is these actions are judged by the perception of the subordinate. It is not uncommon to witness perception that does not mirror reality. This adds a layer of complexity to not only make choices that are, but also appear to be, fair.

The other thought process is the reinforcement theory. Employees behave according to what they think will be outcomes of their actions. Those behaviors that create a good result are rewarded to provide positive reinforcement. Conversely, actions that are not desirable along with their consequences are penalized with negative reinforcement. Supervisors do not have to only provide one type of reinforcement, but rather should use a combination. The distribution of these 2 will shape the culture of the practice. A workplace with only positive responses does not point out, or even try to remediate, deleterious behavior. An environment with only negative reactions can easily become a toxic situation with a detrimental culture and high turnover of employees. The ideal situation is finding the right mix to maximize employee production that is sustainable over a long period of time.

There are many different philosophies a practice can take to reward their employees. One common and successful approach that promotes continued professional growth and hard work is the skills-based pay method. In this environment, employees benefit by seeking out and assuming more responsibilities. This creates additional value in the human resource pool by both widening and deepening its talent.

One particular situation every supervisor should diligently monitor for is staff burnout. Although more common in a practice with a bad atmosphere, employees can still be pressed beyond their limitations. This situation is not only harmful to the individual but also the practice. There are cases that lead to emotional instability, which place that employee, and those around the employee, including family, in an unsafe environment. If there are any suspicions about burnout, it is strongly advisable for the responsible supervisor, or even a fellow coworker, to refer the employee to a wellness program. A company culture that appreciates employee well-being will mitigate this risk.

Immediate Action Items

Is employee turnover an issue in your practice? Do you even know what the turnover rate is? Working with your Human Resources staff, determine not only what the rate is overall, but also break it down to different groups, such as technicians, front office employees, and doctors. Consider why one area is doing better than another and if there is an opportunity for improvement. One question to answer is whether one subordinate style exists in those employees staying longer vs those that leave quickly. If so, you may want to include questions during new employee interviews that would uncover which type the interviewee is to assess his or her compatibility to your system. Alternatively, you can discuss the supervisor's style to see if a different method may result in better outcomes. Successfully reducing the turnover will have many seen and unseen benefits throughout the entire organization. It is worth the time to evaluate and address it.

Navigating Company Dynamics

Importance

Businesses rely on human resources to function by completing tasks on a daily basis. The need for using humans requires the acceptance of the human nature that comes with it. Although the workplace should be a location where work is the only dimension, the reality is that human instinct adds other dimensions to the situation. This complicates the work environment by involving emotions and relationships into routine interactions.[1] These confounding factors, no matter how hard individuals may try to tease them away, play a role in the decision-making process. The repercussions include selecting choices that are not in the best interest of the business but rather for political reasons.

All businesses face the same challenge; however, the leading organizations have methods and staff in place to minimize these influences. The key is to remove emotions and behaviors that are only self-promoting. They should be redirected with actions that unify the team to benefit the organization along with following the vision and mission statements. The goal is to create a response that is consistent with the company culture where the success of the business takes precedent over the individual employee's gains. The hope is that this collaboration still results in an outcome that benefits all parties.

Indirectly, this situation also provides the organization an opportunity to assess which employees truly possess the qualities that align with the greater team goals. The individuals that excel should be empowered. Those that conflict need to be re-evaluated regarding their role in the organization. Set the expectations for employees to behave professionally and in a manner consistent with the desired culture, and then hold them accountable to that performance.

Keywords

Workplace politics: The inner workings and relationships within an organization that influence how it and the employees operate

Scapegoat: An action where the blame of a negative outcome or situation is placed on one or a few individuals that bares the responsibility for the undesired result

Team-building techniques: Various methods used to initiate, develop, and maintain a team-oriented approach

Applications

Workplace politics inevitably affect almost all decisions made in a practice. There is no way of avoiding its influence because its existence is inherent to having human beings as employees. It is a very difficult challenge to completely exclude these considerations for any employee when he or she is in the decision-making process. This stresses the need to recognize that conflict of interest does exist and declare it to maintain transparency. The true test is how to mitigate its impact while implementing a process that remains impartial. What usually accompanies politics is gossip. Unlike workplace politics that cannot be completely removed, effective organizations have a culture where gossip is not tolerated. It only creates more problems and has no value to a practice.

Consider again the example of Beth (Figure 2-3). She has worked alongside Paul, another front office staff member, on many occasions. They interacted so well that Beth introduced Paul to her best friend, Susan. It turns out Paul and Susan dated for a short period of time, but it did not work out. Beth and Paul's relationship has soured since the breakup. Beth and the physician owner of the practice, Seth, are good friends because they knew each other prior to Beth being employed at the practice. Recently, the front office staff received several complaints from other staff and patients about their slow service. Beth pulled Seth aside the next time they saw each. She let him know that all the other front office employees feel they are working hard, but Paul is not meeting his responsibilities. She even comments on how he cannot be trusted and uses him as a scapegoat.

There are 2 responses that Seth can have in this situation. The wrong approach is allowing workplace politics to allow an emotional, knee-jerk reaction to protect a friend in this situation. He directly pulls Paul aside and reprimands him for not working hard. There are multiple problems in this approach, which demonstrate the power of how decision making can be clouded by politics. The first is that Seth allowed Beth to bypass the chain of command from the organizational chart by not initially discussing this with Robyn, her direct report and the Front Officer Manager. This behavior creates a culture that it is ok to circumvent the designed organizational structure. It also voids the trust of Paul towards Seth because the facts were not obtained before a decision was made. It renders Robyn as an inefficient figure head in her role and labels Seth as a hot head.

The ideal response from Seth would have been one of understanding but also redirecting to allow the proper channels to address this issue. Seth could have told Beth the following:

> Thank you, Beth, for sharing your thoughts. I hear your words and want to make sure to address your concerns. It is obvious you care a lot about the practice and our patients. The right next step is to follow our established company guidelines to help

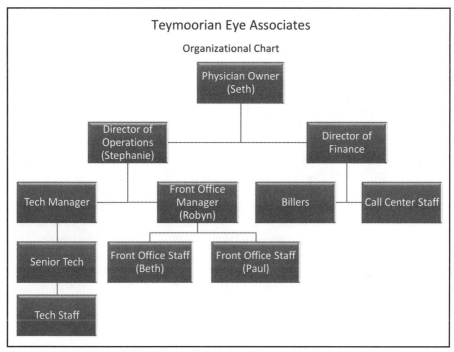

Figure 2-3. Organizational chart illustrating the roles of various individuals.

address this issue in the best manner for all. Have you brought this up with Robyn? I recommend you discuss it with her in order to keep her in the loop and allow her to utilize her experience. If, for some reason, you are uncomfortable with Robyn, then you have safe alternatives to meet with Stephanie or Human Resources.

This approach is empty of politics. It places the interest of the practice ahead of any personal connections. Seth is able to disassociate himself from the situation, which helps maintain a clear, impartial image throughout the organization. He strengthens the credibility of Robyn and reinforces the culture of maintaining the hierarchy from the organization chart. It shows appreciation to Beth's dedication to the practice and provides another route in case her relationship with Robyn has issues. Lastly, it also gives Paul a fair chance to give his account of the situation. This method is not as easy as it goes against a natural, emotional response; however, it provides the best results. Great leaders attempt to recognize all the stakeholders in every situation and then find ways to maximize the benefits for everyone.

One tool that Robyn can use to address this dynamic between Beth and Paul would include team-building techniques. These are implemented to improve and strengthen work relationships. The goal is to increase workers' production and promote a better company culture through positive work environments. Simple examples of these techniques include bridge-building competitions and mine fields. These activities are not limited to companies in trouble but rather can be utilized by healthy practices that are attempting to maintain a positive culture. Successful practices are always receptive to improvement opportunities.

Immediate Action Items

When was the last time your practice had a team-building activity? If there has not been one recently, you may want to consider hosting one. What if everything at the office is great, then should you still invest in an activity? The answer is "Yes" regardless of how the group is performing. These types of exercises benefit all types of interpersonal dynamics from those that are tightly knit to others hanging on by a thread. They focus on core principles and strategies that can be applied over a wide spectrum. The work environment changes over time with employee turnover and as the individuals themselves evolve. The result is a continual stream of new working relationships that everyone needs to navigate. Inevitability, conflict will arise, so having these bonding sessions helps in those instances. They create a safe environment where difficult conversations can occur, which can diffuse hostile situations. For those instances where interactions are strong, the goal is to encourage and further facilitate this interaction. Another benefit is that these activities can incorporate projects that demonstrate the favored company culture.

CRITICAL ORGANIZATIONAL BEHAVIOR POINTERS

* Clear reporting lines are critical to prosperous practices by eliminating many sources of misunderstanding.
* Creating a strong and sustainable organization requires unambiguous direction and goals from leadership.
* The value of great leadership is illustrated by the fact that company culture sets the expectations of employee behavior.
* Successful individuals take time to identify office politics to understand how to react in problematic situations to minimize consequences.
* Understand what type of employee behavior is important, and then base rewards and penalties on those as opposed to encouraging office politics.
* In order to maximize the efforts of employees, the goals of the organization and employees must match.
* Effective organizations understand and appreciate the various managing and subordinate styles of their staff.
* Team-building activities can be a great resource at different times, including the beginning of an endeavor and during times of crises.

* Attempt to keep turnover of employees as low as possible, because there are many hidden negative effects when employees leave and new ones enter, such as the costs of training, loss in productivity, and influence on company morale.
* Do not forget the importance of showing praise and giving thanks to employees for their work because these actions can be viewed to be just as valuable as additional salary.

REFERENCE

1. Robbins SP, Judge TA. *Organizational Behavior*. Washington, DC: Pearson Education, Incorporated; 2017.

3

Maximizing
Human Resources

Human resources isn't a thing we do.
It's the thing that runs our business.

— Steve Wynn

INTRODUCTION

At the end of the day, ocular care is a service-oriented business. This type of work places human beings as a company's most critical investment. Their presence is felt everywhere by playing vital roles in almost all operational processes. These range from the employees that directly interact with patients to those that provide the support needed to effectively execute those tasks. As a result, they represent the most important, yet costly, resource utilized by a business. The responsibility of recruiting, training, and reviewing these human resources falls on the Department of Human Resources (HR). A few applications of HR include implementing annual reviews, mediating in conflict scenarios, handling risk management, and processing payroll.

HR can be an asset that helps a practice excel or a liability that acts like an obstacle. Therefore, the organization of this chapter is a like a game plan for a winning strategy on how to optimize it. The initial focus spotlights the search and acquisition of potential employees. Attention then shifts to training methods for this new personnel. Next, the discussion turns to reviewing and growing them. This transitions into approaches for re-educating and, if needed, terminating those that do not fit the determined standards. It concludes with a section about related but unique topics. This chapter seeks to educate the reader on how to make HR a competitive advantage for the practice as opposed to an expensive expenditure.

Teymoorian S. *Essential Business Fundamentals for the Successful Eye Care Practice* (pp 39-55). © 2019 SLACK Incorporated.

What Is Human Resources?

The most important resource of a business is its human resource—the employees. Whether the goal is to create a valuable good or provide an excellent service, the success or failure of an organization ultimately turns back to the individuals in it. The difficulty is that all businesses are looking for good employees.

The difference between an average organization and a superior one is the ability to get the most out of what is available. The best ones have a commitment and structure in place to locate the right talents, hire the best applicants, provide them the proper training, position them in the most advantageous roles, review and assess their work, and inspire them to grow. This encompasses the roles of HR. The capability to strategically implement HR requires understanding the company's vision, possessing the skill set to effectively manage individuals, and maintaining the proper knowledge about legal rules and regulations.[1,2]

HR also creates some of the most difficult challenges a business faces despite all of its benefits. It is inevitable that organizations will need to deal with employees that do not fit into the overall plans for the future. The reasons for this can significantly vary from structural changes in the business to unacceptable behavior from the individual. Nonetheless, the ability to efficiently transition an employee away is a critical skill. The cost of its inability can be steep with consequences such as a devaluing of the brand, damaging the company culture, and sparking legal action against the business. Forward-thinking organizations understand these repercussions. The goal is to take a proactive approach to prevent these situations rather than a reactive one after an undesirable event occurs.

Human Resources in Eye Care

The value of strategically implementing and utilizing HR in the eye care practice is demonstrated by those organization that always seem to appear bountiful in their exceptionally qualified employees and happy company environment. These elite companies have figured out how to bring in the higher-level applicants despite drawing from the same talent pool as similar competing businesses. However, they do not stop there. Coupled with great leadership, these organizations continue their commitment by creating and fostering a positive work experience that further maximizes their employee potential. They have organized processes to properly position and grow their organization's talent. The important HR abilities to possess in an eye care practice are the following: finding the right applicants, getting the best hires, training the human resources, retaining and evaluating the talent, retraining and releasing employees, and appreciating special human resource topics.

Finding the Right Applicants

Importance

The ability to locate the best applicants to join a company is a measure of how well a business is run. An organization must first understand what their needs are in the job posting to locate the appropriate individuals from a prospective pool. Although employees should be expected to perform their duties, the responsibility of placing employees in the correct position and supplying them the necessary resources to excel falls on the management and leadership team.

Once a company has the necessary HR structure and specifically defined their needs for a particular position, the focus shifts toward identifying the proper personnel. The top organizations align the talent needs requested by leadership with effective strategies to locate and evaluate the appropriate applicants. HR then selects the right individuals to maximize the company's needs through a series of thoughtful interviews and due diligence about the candidates' backgrounds.

Keywords

Human resources: (1) a department within a company that hires, trains, reviews, and terminates employees (denoted as "Human Resources" with capitalized letters or "HR") or (2) the actual human beings that serve as employees (denoted as "human resources" with lower case letters)

Full-time equivalent (FTE): A method to denote the expected work from a hire where this information aids in the measuring of employee production and for allocation of budgets

Job description (JD): A formal description for a position in an organization that provides specifics about its responsibilities and expectations

Resume: The experience, training, and skill set of a perspective employee applying for a position

Communication skills: The ability to listen and respond to others

Open-ended question: A style of question where answers invite detailed responses

Closed-ended question: A style of question where answered require simple responses like "Yes" or "No"

Ability: An employee's aptitude for performing a single or set of tasks

Skills: The composition of an employee's innate and learned abilities

Competencies: The summation of an employee's abilities and skill set

Achievements: A list of accomplished goals that are typically difficult to reach and warrant recognition

Transferable skills: A set of skills that can be used over a wide range of positions with differing job descriptions

Teamwork: The process where a group of individuals work together as a cohesive unit to achieve goals

Body language: The unspoken expressions of emotions and thoughts based on body positioning and behavior

Background check: A review of a potential employee's history for disciplinary action

Reference check: A review of a potential employee's references listed on a job application for accuracy and validity

Applications

The process of successful recruitment is highly dependent on the alignment with the company's leadership team. The desired culture and vision, as described by leadership, must match the individuals that HR is hiring. This required synchrony is not limited to just these large-scale issues; it also trickles down to each individual employee. Usually each hire is referenced to the amount of work that position is expected to produce in terms of a full-time equivalent (FTE). A full-time addition is one FTE, and a part-time is one-half or one-quarter FTE depending on the amount of production expected. This identification keeps track of the employee work amount and budgeting.

The first task in effectively hiring the best candidate is for HR to post a clear job description (JD). This ensures transparency that the position the applicant is looking to fill matches the practice's needs. Otherwise, problems will ensue as soon as the talent is hired. These troubles can extend from poor job performance all the way to legal ramifications if the new hire is required to perform duties that are not listed. An example would be an incorrect description on the amount and type of heavy lifting. There are many JD templates, but it is important to be as accurate as possible. Figure 3-1 is a sample JD for a workup technician.

The next step is localizing those applicants worthy of an interview. The typical response from interested candidates that have reviewed the JD is to submit their resume. HR filters through these resumes to check that the applicant has the appropriate skills and experience to justify an interview.[1] The interview process can range from one to many rounds, including via telephone or in person. Those conducting the interviews, which can be others besides HR, attempt to connect with and understand the candidate. This process tests their communication skills to validate their ability to work with others, including in difficult situations.[3]

Efficient methods include a combination of open- and closed-ended questions with each serving a particular purpose. Open questions provide the candidate an opportunity to show his or her personality by freely answering since these do not have many restrictions. This would include a question such as, "George, can you tell us a little bit about yourself?" Closed questions lead the applicant to specific and focused answers meant to share factual information in a succinct manner. An example would be, "How many years have you been a Certified Ophthalmic Assistant?"

The aggregate responses provide the interviewer the applicant's abilities and skills that help define the scope of the applicant's competencies. The ideal candidate has transferable skills that allow cross-training to other few roles within the practice if called upon. This highlights the importance of teamwork.[1] An advanced interviewer will also examine the applicant's body language to gauge his or her comfort and ability to respond under stress.[3] These reactions represent how the applicant would behave under similar circumstances in the real work environment.

Teymoorian Eye Associates

Job Title: Ophthalmic Technician

Employee Name: _____   **Effective Date:** _____

Full-Time ☒ **Part-Time** ☐ **Exempt** ☐ **Non-Exempt** ☒
Reports To (Position Title): Director of Operations

Summary of Job Purpose: Must be able to check intraocular pressure, conduct manifest refractions, check angles, and acquire accurate chief complaint.

Qualifications: The employee must be willing and able to comply to the criteria of the job description as identified below.

Essential Duties and Responsibilities (other duties may be assigned):
1. Conduct the requirements of an ophthalmic assistant.
2. Monitor tasks in inbox on a routine basis throughout the day.
3. Utilize sound discretion in assisting fellow coworkers.
4. Conduct special projects.
TOTAL:

Supervisory Responsibilities: Yes ☐   No ☒

Education and/or Experience:
- High school diploma or general education degree (GED).

Essential Skills and Abilities:
1. Effective interpersonal interaction and communication
2. Solution oriented with capacity to multitask

Physical Demands:

Lift, Push or Pull	Less than 25%	25% to 50%	Over 50%
Up to 10 pounds		X	
10 to 25 pounds		X	
26 to 50 pounds	X		
51 to 100 pounds	X		

Working Hours: Ophthalmic Technician position requires a working schedule of Monday to Friday from 8 AM to 5PM.

Figure 3-1. Example of a job description for an ophthalmic assistant.

The last step in the process is additional due diligence from HR to conduct both a reference and background check. This crosschecks that the information given by the candidate is accurate and there are no legal concerns that need to be brought up to the practice, respectively. The best time to know these extra details is before hiring the candidate. The consequence of missing this information is a waste of company resources by hiring an individual that does not work out.

Immediate Action Items

Does each position in your practice have a JD? If so, is it updated to include all the activities current employees are performing while listing duties they should also be ideally completing? Review with HR that JDs are accurate, available, and transparent to all current and potential staff members. You never know when a new position will need to be filled in your organization. If it is a critical role, time is of the essence. However, a rushed attempt to find an applicant generally ends in a less than optimal solution. This is due in part to not having the right JD to post and use to screen applicants. The result is a new hire that may not be qualified and not given a clear understanding of what is expected. It typically leads to an even worse situation as now you are left with an employee you need to let go. Not only does that consume valuable time, but firing someone that could not deliver on an inaccurate JD can lead to legal trouble.

If you do not have JDs, then it is time to get them. Either create or modify existing templates to meet the needs of your organization. Make sure that the items listed are correct to give yourself and any employee a fair opportunity to be evaluated and critiqued. The presence of a polished JD also helps separate practices that appear to run well vs those that seem to jump from one fire to another. Prospective applicants, especially great ones, notice the difference.

Getting the Best Hires

Importance

The next critical step is successfully hiring the desired talent that was identified through the interview process. The major challenge encountered at this point is that these applicants can have many potential suitors in the same marketplace. Although skillful HR have the capability to spot overlooked talent that can excel, it is more commonplace to see that other businesses will have noticed the same bright stars.

The leading companies understand the competitive landscape and carefully position themselves to have the best opportunity to land these candidates. They realize that recruitment is actually a 2-way street. The most attractive talents are interviewing the organization as much as they are being evaluated themselves. The ideal recruiter-applicant interaction is one of mutual respect for each other where both understand that a synergistic relationship leads to the best results. The additional yet easily underappreciated benefit to this hiring style is that it demonstrates the true company culture to the candidates.

These types of subtle discussions, along with their tones, separate good from great HR. It makes the difference on either getting or losing those star applicants. The takeaway is that elite businesses have a clear understanding of their identity and culture. They use that information to create a recruitment approach that identifies the applicants that will match easily with it. Once the correct system is in place, it just needs to be used.

Keywords

Suitability: The fit of an employee's ability to a particular need or task for a position in an organization

Compensation: The manner in which an employee is paid for his or her work

Offer: A process in which a prospective employee is given the option to accept the open position in question

Entry-level position: A low-level role in an organization where an employee without much experience first begins in a particular field of work

Sales position: A role in an organization where an employee is part of the sales force

Managerial position: A role in an organization where an employee supervises and manages the activities of those staff members directed to perform duties

Supervisor: An employee that directly oversees the tasks and performance of the individuals below him or her

Manager: An employee that governs the overall priorities of those working under him or her

Director: An employee with an elevated position and responsibility for the overall direction of a given arm within a business (and not the actual execution of the plan, which is left to the supervisors and managers)

Executive position: A high-level role in an organization where an employee with management experience can plan and direct actions on a grand scheme

Chief-Suite (C-Suite): The aggregate of executive-level individuals within an organization

Chief Executive Officer (CEO): The C-Suite individual and highest-ranked employee that has the final say over all matters within a company

Chief Financial Officer (CFO): The C-Suite individual that oversees all financial issues

Chief Operating Officer (COO): The C-Suite individual that governs operations

Chief Informational Officer (CIO): The C-Suite individual that manages the information technology

Chief Medical Officer (CMO): The C-Suite individual responsible for medical matters

Applications

HR proceeds forward to the process of hiring the individual once an applicant passes the suitability test from the interview stage. This stage requires the company to provide the official offer along with its compensation package to the candidate.

Along with many other specifics, the offer defines the type of role the applicant is accepting, which includes entry, sales, managerial, or executive-level. Managerial positions vary depending on the level of responsibility and influence with an ascending order of supervisor, manager, and director. The executive-level is composed of the highest leadership team (C-Suite) including the chief executive officer, chief financial officer, chief operating officer, chief informational officer, and chief medical officer. Not every company, however, will have all of those roles but instead will fill the positions that are needed.

The compensation proposal is a culmination of both external and internal research done by HR. The external component is searching through databases, which can be accessed commercially, to understand the compensation ranges for a similar position in the competitive environment. These numbers are generally fixed since they represent the average of a large aggregate pool. HR takes that information and matches it with the available and desired target amounts from the practice. These numbers are much more dynamic. They will be at peaks when the demand is high or the quality of the applicant is great, or at troughs for the opposite. The result is a proposed package that makes the offer compelling externally but also justified internally.

Immediate Action Items

How comfortable do you feel in being able to properly structure and competitively position your offer to applicants? Some individuals get nervous thinking ahead to any negotiations that may occur. We will deal with negotiations in another chapter, but to successfully position your practice for when that time comes, the initial offer needs to be thought-out and substantiated with evidence. The good news is there are resources to help aid this process. This includes products online and from your respective national ophthalmic or optometric society. Invest in getting this information to become comfortable with what is available. This will provide the necessary groundwork needed to effectively complete this task and strategically initiate the negotiation process by already knowing the competitive landscape.

Training the Human Resources

Importance

The process of hiring the desired applicant does not end once he or she agrees to the company's offer. The next important step is the training and integration of the new hire into the organization's system.[2] This demonstrates the necessity to have comprehensive HR in place that can work to successfully transform the applicant to a fruitful employee. In order for this conversion to be efficient and seamless, there needs to be a thoughtful on-boarding procedure.

Proper assimilation of a new hire requires a team approach to training between HR and the supervisors overseeing the employee. Appropriate integration has both direct and indirect ramifications. Everyone easily understands that the faster a new employee begins to work, the sooner he or she can be productive. What the best companies realize is that the training period is the first real opportunity to demonstrate their culture and set their expectations to the new hire. A better first impression will position the organization in a higher regard with the employee. By taking a longer yet strategic approach initially, this communicates the company's culture that naturally elevates the standard of work expected.

Keywords

Formal training: The official process where an employee in a new role is trained on how to properly perform the expected duties

Job shadowing: The process in which one employee attempts to gain an understanding and perspective of another position by observing other employees in that role

Productivity: The effectiveness of an employee to successfully complete assigned tasks

Time management: The ability to efficiently allot the limited resource of time to accomplish goals

Prioritizing: The ability to order tasks in a fashion in order to first address those with most importance

Multitasking: The ability to properly perform many duties at one time

Applications

The talent is now officially an employee. This is where many common mistakes occur in the hiring process. However, the opportunistic practice uses it as an advantage to separate itself from the crowd. Either due to lack of experience or in haste to have the employee start working, underperforming companies will throw the new hire immediately "into the fire" to be productive. This approach of "on-the-job training" can work, but it is not the right one. It is a costly approach to learn by making mistakes. Not only will this training method require a longer time to get the employee working effectively, but it can also pose legal problems from the practice. These issues can include not providing proper education on the internal workings of the company such as how and when to clock in and out, and external requirements such as HIPAA training.

The better method is to utilize formal training with a new hire. This structured approach provides an efficient pathway to on-board the employee. It ensures that proper training and education are given to fulfill all of the needs to become a valuable member of the team. There can be a particular focus on improving productivity by teaching about time management, prioritizing, and multitasking. This strategic approach benefits the company by maximizing its human resource and the employee by learning essential lifelong skills.

Besides these technical benefits, formal training further demonstrates the positive culture of the practice to the employee. This includes demonstrating the priority of properly equipping its employees with the education to excel in the new environment. The first impression from HR about this organization's culture grounds the employee's perception to a superior level. It also sets the company's professional expectations of the new hire. The exact opposite, including modeling a negative culture, occurs at the practice that does not adequately train. That company is left with the almost impossible task of convincing the new employee later that they are more than just a warm body meant to work. The extra amount and time the company eventually invests into the employee will prove to be futile.

Immediate Action Items

Does your HR department have a formal on-boarding process to help new hires assimilate into the practice and provide the right environment to be successful? The best procedure to bring on new staff comes from the old saying, "Let's not reinvent the wheel." Every company and employees face the same dilemma. One option is to go through numerous iterations to eventually arrive at an efficient method. However, it costs time and money to the organization while frustrating the individual. Instead, look at like-minded practices for their procedures, then utilize the wisdom of your leadership to develop the right plan for your company. For example, engage the Technician Supervisor to list what skills are needed by the new technician to be successful. Other leaders such as the Front Office Director can also be included as some of the tasks performed by the technician may cross over. This approach sets the entire team to win by reducing trial and error time to acquire the necessary skills to be productive.

Retaining and Evaluating the Talent

Importance

One of the hardest challenges any successful organization must face is the constant threat of losing valuable employees to other companies. These businesses can be direct competitors in the same landscape or from other sectors depending on the skill set of the employee. There are instances where the departing employee will have reasons that are impossible to compete with, such as family issues. However, this does not stop the best companies from having strategies in place to improve employee retention.

It is a common misconception that the only factor that influences whether employees leave or stay is financial. Money is important, but a successful plan for retention is deeper. Most individuals new to business underappreciate the soft benefits that play a critical role into employee happiness. Winning organizations appreciate and incorporate these factors daily to mitigate the risk of employee attrition.

A part of keeping employees is the use of evaluation and feedback sections. These activities typically involve both formal and informal meetings that provide opportunities for the company and employees to discuss performance. High-functioning organizations utilize these interactions to continually improve the company while building strong relationships with the employees. It is at the time of possible staff attrition when the strength of these relationships is tested. The difference between average and great business is that the best ones paid attention to these personal interactions before the individual ever thought about leaving.

Keywords

Comprehensive Performance Review (CPR): A formal evaluation process where an employee's performance is evaluated and goals are set for the future

Goals: An expected achievement of an employee based on the role's job description, which is evaluated during the review process

Evaluation: A process where the job performance of an employee is reviewed and rated

Feedback: A part of the evaluation process where an employee's areas of strengths and weaknesses are discussed, along with recommendations for improvement

Performance rating: The scoring of an employee's performance

Performance standard: A metric used to evaluate employee performance that represents the level of expected achievement

Performance efficiency: The effectiveness of an employee's performance relative to a performance standard

Incentive: A bonus for achieving a goal

Succession training: A process in which the needed skill set of a particular position is passed from a superior to a lower-level employee with the goal of one day assuming the higher role

Cross-functional training: A style of training where individuals gain the necessary skills and abilities to perform, not only their own duties, but also those of other team members in different roles

Applications

Effective HR management proceeds to the next stage after the new employee has worked for a period of time. This includes a series of informal conversations where the initial quality of their work is reviewed with the manager. Although these sessions are important to share early thoughts, a formal process is eventually applied through Comprehensive Performance Review (CPR).

CPR provides an official structure to discuss these matters with the employee and appropriate supervisory staff. The inclusion of HR at these meetings varies and depends on the nature of the anticipated discussion. The purpose of a CPR is to provide a professional setting where transparent dialogue is directed toward revisiting goals, performing evaluation, and sharing feedback (Figure 3-2).[3] It is important for the practice to have fair expectations of the employee's work and for the employee to feel he or she will be judged appropriately. There are a plethora of methods to use. A common framework is the use of metrics like performance rating, standard, and efficiency.

Efficient use of CPR benefits both the employee and the practice. Take Ashley, the new technician who was hired 6 months ago at Teymoorian Eye Associates. She meets with Stephanie, the Director of Operations, to have her CPR. The review not only enables Ashley to actively partake in her review, but also provides a method to explain her point of view to Stephanie. This approach enhances employee investment. It also strengthens and supports the desired company culture through

Teymoorian Eye Associates

Comprehensive Performance Review

Employee Name: Ashley _____   **Date of Review:** _____
Director of Operations: Stephanie ____

Performance Rating: 5 = Outstanding, 4= Exceeds Performance Standards, 3= Meets Performance Standards, 2= Needs Improvement, 1 = Requires Immediate Correction

Job Expertise					
Evaluation:	1	2	3	4	5	Feedback:

Quality of Work					
Evaluation:	1	2	3	4	5	Feedback:

Quantity of Work					
Evaluation:	1	2	3	4	5	Feedback:

Consistency					
Evaluation:	1	2	3	4	5	Feedback:

Ingenuity and Drive					
Evaluation:	1	2	3	4	5	Feedback:

Judgement					
Evaluation:	1	2	3	4	5	Feedback:

Cooperation					
Evaluation:	1	2	3	4	5	Feedback:

Temperament					
Evaluation:	1	2	3	4	5	Feedback:

Enthusiasm					
Evaluation:	1	2	3	4	5	Feedback:

Attendance					
Evaluation:	1	2	3	4	5	Feedback:

Performance Efficiency: (Quality + Quantity) /10   **Total Score:**   **Average Score:**

Future Developmental Plans and Goals:_____

Employee Signature: _____   Date: _____

Director of Operations Signature: _____   Date: _____

Figure 3-2. Template of a comprehensive performance review.

professionalism and transparency. The value from this developed culture can be drawn upon if a difficult situation presents at another time.

Stephanie can use this opportunity to review Ashley. Goals are altered depending on Ashley's quality of work. For a positive report, the CPR serves the purpose of encouragement. It provides recognition for excellent work, which can include granting incentives. An additional benefit is to further reinforce the company culture. The discussion pivots to creating new goals for Ashley through a collaboration between the two of them. It lays the groundwork for continued growth, including succession training and cross-functional training.

On the other end of the spectrum, the CPR works as a tool for resetting in cases of negative reports. This discussion is much more difficult to accomplish successfully as the evaluation provided is critical. However, this does not mean that the meeting has to result in a poor outcome. The challenge in this case is for both Stephanie and Ashley to work together to improve Ashley's performance. Stephanie must demonstrate good leadership for this to be successful. She needs to objectively evaluate Ashley's substandard work but also remain supportive. It is Stephanie's responsibility to correctly position and adequately supply Ashley to be productive. Ashley's duty is to acknowledge the feedback and continue her pursuit of improvement through additional feedback. It is not easy to remove the emotions from this meeting, but it is imperative that it be done. A developed culture that sets professional expectations from everyone will aid in that task.

One special point to emphasize is that the CPR can become vital should Ashley continue to not be able to meet her required duties. Careful documentation from the review, including corrective recommendations that were not followed, support the grounds for termination in a legal setting. Practices that do not possess strong HR have a tendency to either not provide proper review or document the troubling behavior. This deficiency can become a major problem should the employee need to be let go.

Immediate Action Items

Is your practice currently performing routine employee reviews? If so, are the number and types of reviews at the optimal amount? The answer to this question will vary depending on the practice. This is determined by how many individuals are employed and the amount of staff available to perform the reviews. The practice should strive to have as many evaluations as possible while not bogging down the administrators that have other duties that need to be attended. However, one formal review should be completed at a minimum and, if possible, a few informal ones done throughout the year. It is easy to fall into the trap of feeling there is no time to do this task. There really will never be an ideal opportunity, but without them, the organization will suffer. This mistake will be magnified if there is a troublesome employee. The practice should be accountable to perform these reviews on a routine basis.

If you are not having reviews, then work with the HR department to select and develop review policies starting from templates that are commercially available. Augment these based upon your practice's needs and goals. Create a list of metrics that are meaningful where the employees can be objectively measured. Remember the saying, "You first must be able to measure it before you can evaluate it." This approach makes it unambiguous and fair to all involved in the process. It also supports the recommendations given for improvement. Like all the other areas of the business, make sure that the measurements used in evaluation encourage and reinforce the favored company culture and goals.

Retraining and Releasing Employees

Importance

There will be cases in all businesses, no matter how great the organization is in terms of HR, where certain employees will not meet the expectations of their duties. These situations are especially challenging to companies because they require delicate personal discussion that can also have legal implications. Extraordinary businesses have strategies and policies in place that excel in these challenging times. This is another example that helps differentiate the average from the best companies. They turn hurdles into opportunities for enhancement.

The initial reaction when faced with substandard employee performance is a series of retraining activities that address the deficient areas. Instead of accepting an employee's poor production and working around these issues, thoughtful organizations look for ways of improvement. They provide methods to identifying these weakness, such as periodic reviews, and chances to remediate them, such as shadowing better performing staff. The takeaway message is that the best companies are always involved in processes that evaluate and grow their human resources. The difference is that there will be a variation of the quality of employees where some will have job growth while others will have skills refined.

Unfortunately, despite the best intended attempts at retraining, some employee relationship will need termination. This decision changes the dynamic between the company and the staff member because the two will now head in different directions. The use of HR is accentuated as this transition can take a negative turn toward legal matters if the process is not handled correctly.[2] Successful organizations have HR along with the necessary infrastructure of documentation and corrective measures in place before an employee is even hired. This allows for a smooth departure for the employee that is respectful and professional.

Keywords

Absenteeism: The repetitive nature of unexcused absence from work

Counseling: A process where a supervisor and employee discuss the employee's behavior and actions with a focus on guidance for the employee on areas of improvement to better achieve goals

Corrective action: A guideline given by a supervisor to an employee as a means to make changes based on evaluations of the employee's performance

Termination: The process where an employee is relieved of his or her duties in an organization because of a particular reason (for cause termination) or without one (without cause termination)

Risk management: A process used to mitigate legal risk of an organization when possible issues may arise

Applications

Consider the situation where Ashley is unable to meet the standards provided by Stephanie or if she exhibits deleterious behavior such as absenteeism. These issues need to be addressed to maintain the professionalism and culture promoted by the practice. Stephanie should proceed to provide counseling and corrective action to fix these issues. This formal and strategic approach ensures that proper measurements are being taken to retrain Ashley to achieve optimum productivity.

If these measures are still unsuccessful, HR needs to consider alternative options. All of the documented activities noted earlier for remediation will help provide the support needed to justify employment termination. These findings are important to the practice because it identifies employees that are not working out as desired. Their value becomes even more evident to aid in risk management should the released employee take legal action. Although it is best to avoid these situations, the time and effort spent by HR helps alleviate these issues. This example reiterates the impact of establishing and maintaining the right company culture. Employees are less likely to pursue legal responses if the culture was positive and valued professional behavior as opposed to one that did not treat employees as important members of the practice.

Immediate Action Items

Does your organization have a structured approach for how to remediate or release an employee if needed? In a room of 100 people, 50 of them will be at or below average for a given skills. It should not be alarming that your practice will face employees that are not performing to expectations. Be prepared for this problem because it will happen. This is where the role of consistent reviews plays a vital part of management. During these evaluations, corrective action to unwanted behavior should be offered and implemented. Discuss with your HR if guidelines are in place for when corrective action needs to be given. Like the other metrics discussed, make sure goals are clear and easily judged. Then, develop an agreed-upon plan with the troubled employee along with a deadline for re-evaluation.

A similar conversation and plan of action needs to be in a place with HR in case the employee does not meet the new expectations. Remember to document all problems and the corrective actions given as it occurs. Dismissing staff requires timely and accurate written data. Also, start the process of vetting a lawyer so your practice will be prepared on where to seek counsel for when an issue arises. Unfortunately, the thought process should not be *if* the organization gets sued but rather *when* it gets sued.

Appreciating Special Human Resource Topics

Importance

At a superficial level, HR can appear to be a hurdle for organizations to move forward by preventing or complicating processes. The reality is that it has the best interest of the business in mind. The overall responsibility of HR is maximizing human talent while keeping the organization away from legal issues.[2] The best businesses appreciate and utilize HR by following Benjamin Franklin's quote of "an ounce of prevention is worth a pound of cure" in their daily interactions and decision making.

One critical task for HR in any organization is to remain up-to-date on relevant laws that pertain to the work environment. This is not an easy job as regulations change consistently. The consequences for not adhering to these laws can be not only significant financial penalties for the business, but also a negative hit to its marketing efforts by damaging its reputation. It is not unusual for these types of private company matters to turn into public news. Successful organizations are trained to use HR for guidance whenever in doubt about how to react in these situations.

Keywords

Discrimination: The unfair treatment of one or a group of individuals based on age, sex, or race

Americans With Disabilities Act (ADA): A law that protects the rights of those with physical and mental disabilities to be granted equal access to jobs and services

Affirmative action: A policy that favors the hiring of individuals from previously discriminated groups

Applications

The many roles of HR include keeping the practice and its policies consistent with new rules and regulations stated by governmental bodies. These laws can affect many different parts of a business. Under the realm of HR, the avoidance of discrimination is especially critical. This covers both employee and patient issues.

One important example is the Americans with Disabilities Act (ADA). ADA stipulates that Ashley, a technician, and Mr. Wilson, a patient, have equal and fair access to be an employee and customer of the practice, respectively. The implications of this include having a wheelchair accessible ramp and methods for communication for individuals with visual or hearing impairment. The takeaway is that the environment must be conducive for all individuals that promotes diversity. Similar to ADA is affirmative action. The top practices, along with their HR, ensure compliance with these policies, allowing them to benefit both internally and externally.

Immediate Action Items

Is the company's HR (along with its leadership team) updated with current laws governing employees and customers? Take a survey to ask their comfort levels in this area. Whether they are educated or not, plan and require routine training for them that can be completed online or at conferences. Document that this is done in case it is ever asked of the practice. Also, ask them if they are properly able to enforce corrective action to the rest of the employees to keep the company compliant with current standards. If there is any hesitancy to this, then carefully modify the practice culture to allow for it to occur. Always remain open to their recommendations even if it is not what you want to hear. They have a tough enough job to bring up unwanted requirements, but they are trying to keep the company out of trouble.

CRITICAL HUMAN RESOURCES POINTERS

* The first step in proper recruiting or promoting of an employee is to have a clear JD that matches the needs of the organization.

* It is unrealistic to set expectations for employee improvement if a proper review of the employee's work is not provided along with achievable and defined milestones.

* Do not create positions or JDs because of the skill set of one employee, but rather define the position that is needed and look for appropriate candidates for the job.

* The most expensive costs in an organization are human resources. Invest time and resources into them so you can get the most from your investment.

* The successful practice is able to recruit, train, and keep talented individuals, which not only provides better customer care, but can also decrease costs by maximizing employee efficiencies.

* Maintaining proper employee records, including corrective and disciplinary actions, is critical in risk management.

* Although it may appear at times that HR simply gets in the way of a business, its main responsibility is keeping the business out of legal trouble while helping to optimize employee performance.

* It is always better to alert HR about risk management early as opposed to waiting and hoping a bad situation will improve by itself.

* Strong HR remains up-to-date with new regulations, so use that knowledge to strategically compete in your playing field to acquire and retain the best talent.

* In certain cases of human resources, the departure of a suboptimal or toxic employee is better for an organization, which leads to the thought of "addition by subtraction."

REFERENCES

1. Yate M. *Knock 'em Dead: Hiring the Best*. Avon, MA: Adams Media, Incorporated; 2014.
2. Armstrong S, Mitchell B. *The Essential HR Handbook: A Quick and Handy Resource for Any Manager or HR Professional*. Wayne, NJ: Career Press; 2008.
3. Covey, S. *The 7 Habits of Highly Effective People*. New York, NY: Simon & Schuster, Incorporated; 2013.

4

Optimizing Operations

The art of simplicity is a puzzle of complexity.

— **Douglas Horton**

INTRODUCTION

Eye care providers appreciate the importance of properly following procedures in an organized fashion to achieve the best results. These procedures represent a process. A classic example is refraction. The study of operations is the application of these processes in a business. It transforms the abstract company goals into concrete procedures with a carefully choreographed order of steps. Each planned step efficiently utilizes the available valuable resources to complete the given task. The process is then analyzed for waste, improvements are made, and the cycle starts again.

Many processes occur around the practitioner all day. Most go unnoticed because they have been maximized through trial and error over a long period of time. The most common procedure encountered in a practice is the patient experience. This includes all the steps taken from the moment a patient enters and leaves the office. However, many sub-processes must have been completed to make that patient encounter successful. A procedure was used to create the doctor's template for when patients scheduled appointments. All of the staff members who interacted with the patient, from the front office to the technicians, went through training that involved a series of educational modules. The eye drops used to anesthetize and dilate the patient's eyes were part of an inventory process to make sure they were available for use when needed.

Teymoorian S. *Essential Business Fundamentals for the Successful Eye Care Practice* (pp 57-70). © 2019 SLACK Incorporated.

To exemplify the theme of operations, this chapter will take a step-by-step approach to demonstrate the procedures on optimizing the many processes that surround us every day. It begins with an introduction to different process types and how they create the targeted purpose. The next step includes the methods used to assess the various steps and the overall procedures. This leads to strategies on identifying and changing the problem areas that create inefficiencies in the system. The culmination of these topics results in a systematic approach on how to continually improve the processes through an effective and repeatable cycle.

WHAT IS OPERATIONS?

Businesses are judged by the value of the final products created or the services provided. However, for each product or service that is sold to consumers, companies must first create and follow a series of steps in a process.[1] The method used to perform these procedures have a significant impact on the end products. These include the cost of making the product, the time needed to create it, and the quality in which it is produced.

The inherent variability in these steps presents an opportunity. An elite company understands each step and how they are linked together from the beginning to end. This enables a productive cycle of continual evaluation and improvement for the critical processes in an organization. This procedure is strengthened when it aligns with the goals, mission, and overall vision of the business.[1]

Each company's ambition should be to reach a level of process development where sustainable quality improvement is achieved. This occurs when each step is carefully examined and reviewed with the purpose of making changes that lead to incremental refinement. Achieving that high functional status in an organization is actually a process in itself. The initial step includes appreciating the variations that exist between and in each business. This realization illustrates the importance of flexibility when designing different processes based on needs.

The system is then permitted to function after selection of the process type. At the same time, evaluations are made using carefully guided metrics that produce reliable data to be analyzed. This information tags weak areas for improvement. The process then repeats itself for further examination and enhancement. Each step should ensure the pathway being taken is in alignment with the targeted business goals as the process becomes more refined. This exercise provides a strategic advantage to those companies that learn to adapt and improve themselves. In stark contrast, there will be other organizations that are content with being stagnant but will eventually find themselves obsolete.

OPERATIONS IN EYE CARE

The impact of operations for an eye care business is witnessed by taking a moment at the workplace to watch the employees carry out their duties. Everything being done is part of a process to accomplish a goal. All similar businesses perform the same activities. However, they greatly differ in efficiency. This is what separates great from average practices. The opportunistic companies realize this variability to create a meaningful advantage. They take time to fundamentally understand each step. They acquire knowledge that leads to the creation and implementation of a review process. This allows for perpetual improvement on the overall system while remaining optimal despite changing conditions. The fundamental competencies in operations for the successful eye care practitioner to possess are understanding process types, implementing process development, incorporating evaluation and metrics, and identifying problems and improving processes.[1]

Understanding Process Types

Importance

Once a business has direction as described through its vision and mission statements, it needs to develop and exercise a plan on how to achieve these goals. The focus shifts to the practical applications of operations. The critical tasks at this junction are to identify and select a business model, then it needs to implement processes throughout the organization to facilitate the execution of this strategy. Thriving organizations efficiently execute the tasks required to convert their big dreams into reality.

The first difficulty is the selection of the correct model for implementation. The best approach on how to choose the right model, and its associated processes, is to remember the characteristics and goals of the organization as a whole. In the ideal setting, there is strategic alignment throughout the business. Each step along the journey builds on the prior one. The vision for the business outlines its mission. This, in turn, guides the model that leads the processes. The intended organizational culture acts as a safety check along the pathway to ensure quality control. When these different sections work in unison, a fundamentally strong and talented company exists that is primed to thrive.

Keywords

Operations: A discipline of business that focuses on the creation, utilization, and improvement of processes in a company

Process: The cumulative step-by-step procedure of creating a good or providing a service

Business model: A concept that is structured with guidelines on how to run the operations of a business

Business plan: The way in which a business model is executed

Process map: A description explaining the relationship of steps in a process
Outsourcing: The use of an outside entity to provide a necessary a step or an entire process in operations

Applications

The ability to run an eye care practice effectively is contingent on orchestrating a plethora of interwoven steps together to create a masterpiece of operations. Each of these steps represents a process. These processes contribute a part to the whole, with some being more essential than others. There are many benefits to this structured creation. It can be broken down to smaller sections, analyzed for efficiencies, reconfigured if needed, and then put back into its original position. The elite practices understand how each process functions and appreciate its individual value.

The blueprint for directing these activities is explained by the practice's business model. It furnishes the intended structure and goals to be viewed at the 30,000-foot level. An example would be the creation of a large, multi-specialty eye care practice that provides excellent patient care. This includes maximizing economics of scale both medically by having many subspecialties and financially by employing the optimal number of providers. The finished products created by the business model should align with the company's vision and mission statements. These fundamental components provide the pillars on which the desired culture rests.

The business plan outlines the steps required to execute these directives. It utilizes process maps to demonstrate the proper sequences of the individual segments. A sample would be to create and use an intricate organizational chart that provides leadership in key positions of the practice, such as Director of Operations and Director of Finance.

The best companies also realize there will be instances where the practice would be better off by allowing an outside expert entity to provide a step or an entire process. This is accomplished by strategic outsourcing. An extreme example of this would be outsourcing Human Resources or Information Technology from a practice to another professional company that specializes in those areas.

Immediate Action Items

Have you ever considered what one of your patients experience during a typical examination at the office? Does this match with your desired business model? The patient experience process is the most important of all the ones that take place as it represents your source of income and influences the ability to provide patient care. Take a moment to diagram out a routine appointment that represents what you think is the patient flow. Show that figure to several staff members and ask for their input to refine the sequence as you may not have subtle events that occur. If there is anything missing that you believe should be there or removed, take note of it. Keep this diagram as we work through this chapter together. The good news is we only have positive progress to make as we carefully evaluate and refine this important process in your practice.

Implementing Process Development

Importance

The ability to effectively execute a business model depends on the quality of processes that are utilized to achieve the goals. The benefit of understanding process management is the opportunity to customize each step to fit the needs of individual tasks throughout an organization. It provides different areas of a business the capacity to alter steps, which enables continuous assessment and subsequent improvement. Strong organizations capitalize on this flexibility to maximize production through the best use of their resources. This drives efficiency throughout the business that results in better outcomes for both the company and its customers.

The general strategy used for process management includes a series of steps that create, analyze, and refine its operations. A frequent mistake is the requirement to develop the perfect process the first time and have it completed before it is ever put into use. It is important to think ahead about what the best process would be to use. However, it is very uncommon to have all of the necessary information before starting a process. At some point, the first step needs to be taken. It should be done with the understanding that there will be the opportunity to fine-tune it later to improve its efficiency. The alternative to this option is to never initiate a process, but then nothing will ever be implemented. This leaves the organization with an undesirable label and culture of being static as opposed to adaptable with the changing environments.

Keywords

Logistics: The planning, managing, and executing of each step in a process

Critical path diagram: An algorithm that depicts how the order of steps in a process can be arranged with the goal of best optimizing time

Backward pass analysis: A critical path diagram evaluation that estimates time on the basis of when steps can occur at the latest moment without interfering with the timing of a process

Forward pass analysis: A critical path diagram evaluation that estimates time on the basis of when steps can occur at the earliest times to complete a process

Gantt chart: A schematic used to illustrate when each part of a process will start and end relative to each other

Idle time: An inefficient or wasted period of time in a process when available resources can do work but do not have the necessary materials to complete the step

Bottleneck: The rate-limiting step in a process

Lead time: A quantity of time needed before a required step or process can be initiated

Downtime: A time when either a step or the entire process cannot occur for a particular reason

Forecasting: An exercise in predicting the future based on historical data

Variability: An inconsistent or unpredictable quality of something

Bullwhip effect: A phenomenon that demonstrates inefficiencies in supply chain management based on forecasts of demand where the effects are most noted later in a process

Applications

All eye care practices utilize processes to achieve goals. However, the best organizations do not just deal with these procedures, but rather they thoughtfully perform logistics. Logistical application goes beyond simply lining up steps to compete a process. It requires intimately understanding each step. This includes both internal and external factors. For example, there needs to be appreciation of all the critical subcomponents that must first be aligned for successful completion of that step. There also has to be an awareness of how that particular step influences its counterparts in the overall process.[1]

Successful companies critically assess their processes with a few objectives in mind. They maximize resources to produce the highest-quality product and services while existing in a fluid workspace. A classic example in eye care are all the steps taken from the moment a patient checks in and eventually checks out of an appointment. Every individual practice will have efficient and inefficient ways of performing this duty. However, there is no one cookie-cutter way to approach this problem. This exists due to constant environmental variation, such as changes in the number of technicians available on a given day or for an extended period of time.

The first step to effectively integrate logistics involves understanding how processes are created along with their basic characteristics. This proceeds with diagramming the steps and their required order needed to complete every task. One method utilizes the creation of a critical path diagram that organizes this process with the goal to minimize completion time. Additional information from this diagram can be obtained by performing a backward and forward pass analysis that would detail how late or soon each step can occur without interfering with the system, respectively. This provides insight on how each segment is interconnected with others. Other methods exist to accomplish this task, such as a Gantt chart.[1]

These evaluations focus on decreasing or eliminating idle time. There can be several reasons for this wasted time, but there are a few common sources. Although some causes are unavoidable, it does not mean they cannot be minimized. The first is the presence of a bottleneck. The bottleneck is the rate-limiting step in a process similar to chemical reactions taught in general chemistry. The whole process can only go as fast as the bottleneck will allow. Options to improve its rate are to add more capacity at that step, divert any unnecessary work done at that time to another step, or position it elsewhere.

Consider the patient flow through Teymoorian Eye Associates. All patients seeing the glaucoma specialist receive a visual field test on the same day before seeing the doctor. However, this step is the longest in the process. The doctor can only see as many patients as visual fields can be performed. The cost of the physician is much more than that of the visual field, so there are wasted resources. Solutions to this problem would be to add more visual field machines or not have all patients perform a visual field on every visit. On further analysis, the visual field technician is also refracting the patient to use the correct prescription during the test. Therefore, there are instances when the machine is not in use despite being the slowest step. The refraction task can be separated out and performed by another technician to keep the visual field machine working at all times.

Another cause of wasted resources is lead time. Imagine a different scenario at the practice. The demand from retina patients is overwhelming the specialist despite working at capacity. The practice decides to hire another retina doctor to address the demand. However, it will take 4 to 6 months in lead time before the new physician can start. The company needs to post the position, interview and hire the doctor, give notice to the prior practice, and then complete the on-boarding process. The ideal solution to minimizing this time is proper preparation and anticipation that such a demand may develop. The best practices already have their physician hiring processes in place that minimizes the time needed for when it is called upon to execute. Human resources, marketing, and operations are all prepared for that challenge.

The other reason for idle time is downtime. In any process, there are instances when certain steps are stopped for maintenance or are nonfunctional. For example, a practice's electronic medical record application will be down while its software is upgrading. The easiest answer is to install the upgrade after working hours. If that is not possible, the practice can elect to revert to paper records and then convert those encounters to electronic when the system is back running. However, if that also cannot be done, the practice can anticipate this downtime and minimize staff to only the essential core. This will prevent incurring unnecessary employee costs that will go unused.

The preceding examples hint at the need of anticipating what might be required ahead of time to start preparation for a change in demand. This falls under the category of forecasting in operations. The need for predicting and planning is that variability in a system adds to its complexity. Not properly addressing these deviations leads to inefficiencies and lost opportunities.

Consider the changes in patient volume throughout the year. For a given practice, history reveals lows in January and May but peaks in August and December. There are several reasons for this variation. These can differ from one practice to another depending on changes from internal and external forces. The key is to strategically anticipate these disparities to maximize resources. During low periods, it may be useful to allocate vacation time for idle staff like front office personnel or technicians. This changes during times of higher demand when office hours might be extended or seasonal staff can be hired.

One related finding important to note and be aware of is the bullwhip effect (Figure 4-1). It occurs when subtle variations throughout a process continue to magnify and result in large forecasting errors near the end. For example, consider the following case where patient demand is expected to rise in December.

It is the end of the year, so patients want to come in to use their insurance, and their children who also need exams are home from school. The Director of Operations attempts to determine the appropriate staffing to meet this need and arrives at a conclusion. If there will be more patients wanting to be seen, there should be more staff in the call center to triage the increased call volume. The scheduled patients from these extra appointments will eventually present to the office, so there should be more front office staff. However, slightly more staff will be allocated to work at that time to avoid a shortage in the front office. The additional staff will process more patients, so there will need to be more technicians. It is better to have

Figure 4-1. The Bullwhip Effect.

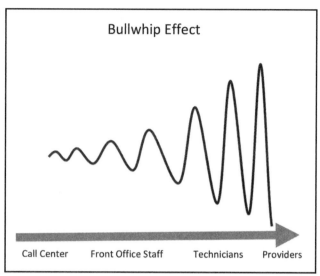

a surplus rather than a shortage of technicians similar to the issue with the front office. Therefore, there will be slightly more technicians than needed. This thought process continues down the pathway until it reaches the physicians. At this point, the magnification of variance between expected and actual is so high that the chances for error are great. The result is miscalculated staff and wasted resources. This exercise stresses the importance of minimizing variability as much as possible and not straying off a projected path to account for unjustified thoughts.

Immediate Action Items

Is the bottleneck in your patient flow process optimized? Advise your staff that you will be assessing the patient flow through the office. To provide an understanding of what is occurring and where improvements can be made, require the staff to document the start and stop time for every interaction they have with a patient. The number of interactions should match the patient flow diagram that was created earlier in the chapter. Gather the recorded information and analyze it to identify where the bottleneck exists. Obtain from HR the cost of each staff member for each part of the process. Is your bottleneck the most expensive part and working at 100% utilization? It is common for this to be the doctor's exam. If it is not, then your process is underutilizing its resources. Let's continue with this example as the chapter progresses to figure out how to enhance this process.

Incorporating Evaluation and Metrics

Importance

The next step in process utilization is performance efficiency assessment. There are many methods to evaluate processes. The most important takeaway to this section is that it occurs in your practice. Once companies and their associated processes are up and running, there is a tendency to get so caught up in other areas that a review of its processes never happens. The trouble with either being unaware or delaying this analysis is that wasteful activities and suboptimal results will continue until they are addressed. Productive businesses allocate resources for continual learning to improve on their current processes by using well-devised metrics. Not only does this behavior keep them efficient, but it also forces them to remain current with the happenings in the competitive landscape.

Keywords

Metrics: A measure in which output is evaluated

Benchmarking: An analysis where the performance of a process is compared to a standard

Flow time: The length of time needed for one thing to go from the beginning to the end of a process

Cycle time: The length of time from the end of having one thing being completed in a process to the next thing being finished

Capacity: The highest output that can be achieved in a particular process over a certain time without any constraints on the pathway

Throughput: The amount of output a process can achieve in a set period of time

Takt time: The actual cycle time or the inverse of throughput

Utilization: A metric that describes how efficiently a process is being used and defined as the ratio of throughput over capacity

Queue: A line created at a step in a process waiting to proceed forward

Wait time: The time spent at a step in a process waiting to proceed forward

Line balancing: A strategy in which certain steps in process are combined or separated to decrease individual idle time by matching the time through the bottleneck step

Applications

Before changes to a process can be made, proper measurements must be taken on its performance. This illustrates the importance of having thoughtful and correct metrics in any procedural set. The values from these indices can then be compared to averages in the same industry through the process of benchmarking. This assessment provides a sense of how well the process is doing and demonstrates to what degree they need to be altered if changes are needed.

There is a set of common metrics that can be applied to most processes. For example, imagine that an eye care practice is evaluating its patient flow procedure. For the sake of simplicity, there is only one of each of the following resources, along with its associated amount of time needed to complete it: front office receptionist (3 minutes), technician (12 minutes), practitioner (10 minutes), and back office biller (2 minutes). Also, the receptionist and the biller use the same computer, and it takes 1 minute to change from the computer program one uses to the other.

The measured time can be converted to metrics that will then allow for benchmarking to look for areas of improvement. The flow time for a patient to go from beginning to end is 27 minutes. The cycle time, which starts when the first patient leaves to when the second patient exits, is 28 minutes. The extra minute is due to changing computer programs from biller to receptionist. The office is open for 4 consecutive hours in the morning, so its capacity is 8 patients. However, the throughput is measured at 7 patients in that time span because of how the operations are organized. The takt time is 34 minutes based on the actual throughput of patients in 4 hours. The result is a utilization of 88%. In real life, these processes are much more complex as there are many different combinations and permutations that can exist. The principles remain the same. Strategic advantages arise from examining the situation and evaluating for improvements to help optimize the process.

Another layer of difficulty to this evaluation is that more than one customer can accumulate at a given step. This results in the creation of a line or queue at a given step in the process. The queue is viewed as wait time for the customer. One common challenge in every successful practice related to this is to decrease the perceived wait time for patients.

There are 2 approaches to consider when addressing this queue problem. First, effective practices attempt to improve their operations to decrease the objective wait time. This includes applying review methods that permit continual measurement, analysis, and change. These approaches will be discussed in the next section. However, one common strategy to reduce wait time is that of line balancing. The case given before about bottlenecks and the visual field step exemplify this method. The refraction duties were transferred elsewhere from the bottleneck position occupied by the visual field technician. The key is to have a true understanding about what is being done and needs to be accomplished in each step. This enables a careful assessment of how it can be altered based on available resources to reduce the bottleneck.

Second, successful companies employ tools to minimize the subjective wait time. Similar to amusement parks, customers in a queue benefit from knowing how long they should expect to be in a particular step. The eye care practice can use this method by telling the patient about how long the wait is for the next part of the process. A typical statement would be, "Ms. Smith, now that we are done taking your images, Dr. Teymoorian should be with you in the next few minutes." If the wait time is expected to be longer, then it is important to update the time by saying, "Dr. Teymoorian is in the middle of laser procedure and should be with you in about 15 minutes."

Also, if a patient has been at one step for a period of time, it is important to acknowledge the wait and attempt redirection. An example would be, "Sorry for the delay as we wait for the visual field machine to open. In the meantime, can I get you some water or a magazine?" It is important to update the patient before the patient asks to be updated. The former shows a sense of caring while the latter makes the company look overbooked.

Another technique incorporates methods to keep customers busy while waiting. The common solutions are television and magazines. However, it is important to be kept updated with the trends of the targeted audience and their associated customer profiles. An example includes the addition of Wi-Fi to the office to enhance the use of personal electronics. All of these approaches help to manage the perceived wait time. As a side note, forward-thinking practices will first direct customers that log on to the network to the practice's landing page on its website. This complements marketing efforts by improving search engine optimization. These elite businesses always ask if processes can be changed to create improvements including to areas that may not be readily apparent.

Immediate Action Items

How good is your patient flow process vs other practices? More importantly, can you be doing it better? You have already completed the first steps with diagraming out your process and then measuring time for each step. Time is one metric, but it is usually the most standard and universal one to start with in this review. It can be used to calculate many essential numbers like flow time, capacity, and utilization. You now know how the length of time one patient takes for his or her whole encounter, how many patients can be seen in each period time, and how efficiently your system sees patients. This information will provide you with an understanding of how your practice is running by viewing it through different lenses. To get a sense of how you compare, benchmark to standards that are available online or from your ophthalmic society.

Think about what metric is important to your practice specifically. Some common responses are the rates of conversion to advanced intraocular lenses from surgical counselors to the cost of glasses sold per optician-patient encounter. Additional metrics in these areas consider not just the amount of time spent, but rather the revenue generated per minute spent. In other words, it would be more beneficial for a practice to have an optician sell $800 in glasses over 30 minutes vs $100 over 15 minutes. Although time is important, make sure to take in other relative metrics that would make your consideration change as to whether a step in a process is effective. Then, benchmark to other practices to help with comparison, such as the prior example with time by itself. Also, additional useful metrics can be found along with your benchmarking search that you may have never considered using.

Identifying Problems and Improving Processes

Importance

The last step in this cycle is to incorporate the analysis results to create positive change. This requires strategic utilization of the information gathered through metric application from the previous section. A common mistake of businesses is the attempt to change processes but doing so without the support from measured data. This makes decision making a guessing game on what to do instead of logically selecting the best option. There are times when guessing works because even a broken clock is right twice a day. However, businesses that make decisions on guesswork place themselves at serious risk for failure. Winning organizations obtain the best information so they can arrive at answers that provide the highest chance to be correct.

Keywords

Value-added (VA): An expenditure of a resource during a process that increases the value of the product or service

Non–value-added (NVA): A wasted expenditure of a resource during a process that does not increase the value of the product or service

Waste: An inefficient use of valued resource

Business–value-added (BVA): An expenditure of a resource during a process that does not increase the value of the product or service but does provide benefit to the business and its processes

Define-Measure-Analyze-Improve-Control (DMAIC) process: A series of steps used to evaluate and improve a process

Fishbone diagram: A cause-and-effect schematic representation that lists all possible sources of error that can help identify the problem with the hopes of localizing the causative issue

Applications

Effective operations management requires a thorough evaluation of the value provided by each step in a process. Although it is important to seek maximization at every level, the first assessment should be if the step is value-added (VA). These create measurable value to the process. Non–value-added (NVA) steps should be eliminated as they generate waste. This does not mean that those that do not create direct financial value are not necessary. There are certain steps that are business–value-added (BVA) by playing an integral part in completing the process. Consider a patient sent to an oculoplastic specialist for evaluation of drooping eyelids. A VA step is the use of billed visual field test to assess effects on peripheral vision. An evaluation of color vision is NVA as it serves no relative purpose for the consulting reason. A BVA step is the measurement of margin reflex distance because it is critical in the diagnosis and treatment for blepharoplasty.

The best practices consider this evaluating exercise as part of a larger process for sustained improvement. The utilization of a continuous method that results in subtle changes allows the business to remain effective in a changing landscape. One particular method is the Define-Measure-Analyze-Improve-Control (DMAIC) process.[1] The protocol for this application follows its name.

* Step 1: The situation and its goals are identified, including the problem and its targets.
* Step 2: The process is allowed to run, but thoughtful measurements using metrics are taken.
* Step 3: The information gathered is analyzed, such as with the use of a fishbone analysis, and benchmarked for effectiveness.

* Step 4: The procedures identified to provide functional improvement are instated.
* Step 5: The positive results are controlled to ensure sustainability for the new processes.

This exercise can be applied to the call center that triages phone calls for an eye practice. For example, there is a problem of excessive dropped calls that go unanswered. This results in poor customer service and a decrease in patient volume. Measurements of employee performance are taken to gauge the current situation and understand its scope. This includes the volume and length of the calls answered. The results are analyzed by comparing them to benchmarks and evaluated for areas of weakness. One issue noted was the lack of proper knowledge from the employees about the services provided and how to triage into the providers' schedule. This forced the call center staff to connect with the technicians in the office to answer the questions. The solution to this problem was regular, formal training for the entire staff about the services offered in the practice. To ensure sustained results, the call center employees are routinely tested about their knowledge and provided adjunctive education to supplement deficient areas.

Immediate Action Items

Are there steps in your patient flow process that are underperforming? If so, you have completed one of the most important steps in any process—you recognize that there is a problem. All businesses have the same issues, but the best ones know how to identify them, make changes, and reassess the situation. There are several different methods available such as DMAIC, each with their strengths and weaknesses. We have already completed the first few steps with our working example from the prior sections. The next step is to take your patient flow process and make changes based on the inefficiencies you have identified. Once the appropriate alterations are made, you should give the practice time to start following it. Then, re-examine the situation again just as you did the first time and localize weaknesses. Repeat this procedure over and over. Not only will this help in improving the process, but it will also give you a valuable understanding of all the critical steps along with their interdependencies.

If you do not have underperforming steps, I recommend you change your focus on how to keep your processes working efficiently. Do not become complacent with your success and feel that change is never needed. It is beneficial to intermittently reassess your practice to ensure that things are working properly. This is why airplanes have routine maintenance check. It is easier to catch a potential problem than deal with the repercussion once one exists, along with its downstream consequences.

CRITICAL OPERATIONS POINTERS

* Take time to understand the company's goals in order to develop processes that align with them.
* The process of continual evaluation and improvement allows a business to remain flexible with the changing environment it lives in.
* Attempt to incorporate and use metrics to not only evaluate an entire process but also each step to identify waste.
* Search for benchmarks in the industry when you are unsure of what metrics to use or expectations to have for a given process.
* Try to minimize variability as much as possible to allow for better forecasting.
* Just because a step in the process does not create value to the customer does not mean it can't add value to the business. Identify and appreciate the value of BVA.
* Improving the perception of wait time can have a significant effect on a patient's impression of the quality of service.
* Identify the costlier steps in your processes and maximize utilization of them; the doctor should not be sitting idle in the office.
* Critically assess the bottleneck in a process to determine if it can be unbundled to make the overall operation more efficient.
* If the takt time is greater than the cycle time in a process, inefficiencies exist; evaluate to see if changes are feasible and worthwhile.

REFERENCE

1. Kamauff J. *Manager's Guide to Operations Management*. Madison, WI: The McGraw-Hill Companies, Incorporated; 2010.

5

Applying Economics

Economics is a social science, not a physical science.

— Jim Stanford

INTRODUCTION

Everyone's life, including that of a practitioner, is filled with examples of economics and its governing principles. We live in world where goods and services are often limited. No one person possesses all of them. This situation necessitates trade among individuals to obtain the right resource mixture. Most exchanges occur without us understanding or appreciating the core theories behind them. However, the outcomes of these barters play a critical role in the health of a business. Naïve strategies used during exchanges lead to suboptimal outcomes.

Economics is really a game between 2 teams—the suppliers and the demanders. The primary medical example most people associate with this is the supply of doctors to the demand of patients. A deeper look into this study reveals its wider application all around us. For example, providers can play on one side or the other depending on the circumstances. On one hand, they supply goods like glasses and services like refractions. On the other hand, they demand goods like hardware needed for electronic medical records and services like maintenance of their visual field machine. The successful eye care practitioner sees this as an opportunity and applies fundamental gameplay strategies to win in each situation.

Teymoorian S. *Essential Business Fundamentals for the Successful Eye Care Practice* (pp 71-84).

This chapter navigates the reader through a process that explains fundamental economic principles and its uses in eye care. Initially, the discussion lays the groundwork with the topics of microeconomics and macroeconomics. The attention turns to resource exchange principles. These develop further with examinations into how resources are accounted for and produced. The goal of this chapter is to equip the practitioner with the essential skill set of identifying when these economic situations occur and how different parties behave to obtain these valued resources.

What Is Economics?

Business exists because there are individuals who possess a resource and others that desire it. Those that wish to have it are willing to give up something of equal or greater value in exchange for it. This describes the basic rules of economics. The best owners understand this relationship and strategically position their organizations to excel when these opportunities present themselves.

Certain economic laws are derived from the interactions between suppliers and demanders. The correct application of these principles has a major impact on the prosperity of a business. Consequently, a lack of economic understanding leads to costly errors. Two frequent mistakes based on common misconceptions, for example, exemplify this issue. The first is that always producing more product will translate to greater profits. This is incorrect as situations exist where each additional unit hurts the business. The second is that the total cost associated with a product simply equals the money needed to buy the necessary parts to build it. In actuality, the determination of cost is much more complex as there are many other considerations. The takeaway is recognizing when these assumptions are inaccurate and correcting for them. The right thought process leads to the best decisions and better results.

Economics in Eye Care

The importance of comprehending and applying economic principles in eye care is illustrated by how practitioners go about procuring the required resources for their practices.[1] In an era when profit margins are diminishing like in medical reimbursements, the ability to efficiently obtain and effectively utilize scarce resources becomes magnified. The ideal method to optimizing the relationship between a supplier and a consumer is to understand how basic principles of economics work. These lead to successful applications in different scenarios. Beyond those rules that dictate supply and demand, additional strategies on various aspects in this area can be applied. The fundamental wisdom in economics for the eye care practitioner to demonstrate are the following: understanding micro- and macroeconomics basics, appreciating supply and demand, minimizing cost, maximizing price, and optimizing scale.

Understanding Micro- and Macroeconomics

Importance

The core principles that businesses are built upon remain constant across all types and areas. What makes them and the marketplaces they work in different from one to the other are the assets involved in the transactions. The thought processes used and theories applied are the same. Successful individuals and organizations use an efficient methodology along with their experiences to obtain maximum results in these interactions.

Keywords

Economics: The study of how scarce resources are utilized in society

Scarcity: The condition that resources are limited in nature

Microeconomics: The study of how individual units or groups make use of resources and their interaction in markets

Macroeconomics: The study of how resources are used throughout an entire economy

Recession: A period of time when there is a reduction in the economy usually associated with a decline in gross domestic product

Gross domestic product (GDP): The value of all goods and services produced in a given period

Import: A good produced outside of a nation but sold within it

Export: A good produced inside of a nation but sold outside of it

Applications

Economic principles and applications govern the practitioner's interactions with others, including patients, staff, vendors, and even family and friends. They exist because no one person possesses all the resources needed to function. Instead, individuals use trade to exchange one resource for another. This relationship becomes complex because the abundance of these resources can significantly vary from one to another. Therefore, each resource has a different value. Those with more scarcity have greater value relative to abundant ones.

These exchanges between individuals or small groups are categorized under microeconomics. For example, consider the situation where Teymoorian Eye Associates is looking to hire a new biller for the finance department. The practice is willing to exchange resources in the form of salary and compensation to acquire the time and skill set of a qualified applicant. The relative abundance of the job opportunities to the number of those seeking the positions will determine the fair market price in this situation. If there are more applicants than jobs, a lower salary can be offered as opposed to a situation where there are more jobs than applicants that would necessitate a higher salary.

However, these interactions are not restricted to those only involving a few individuals. Similar principles apply on a larger scale including between countries.

These cases fall under macroeconomics. This does not mean that macroeconomic exchanges do not affect small groups. A single person still works in an environment influenced by the larger dynamics of a country.[2] Issues like inflation and recession affect the provider's daily practice. Additional topics such as gross domestic product and its affiliation with imports and exports also play a role. Successful practitioners understand these rules and their consequences. They then apply them in the decision-making process when applicable to make the best choices.

Immediate Action Items

In what marketplace does your practice reside? The simple answer is eye care. However, you need to carefully contemplate the question and be very specific about your answer. This is essential because, as you will see throughout the text, each chapter requires a clear understanding of who your company is and what it does exactly. Also, is this the correct marketplace you should be in or is there a better one that deserves to be considered? This will be addressed later as the subject matter needs to be built upon to answer it.

So, what exactly does your practice provide as a resource? For example, some offer a high-end premium experience that tailors to those having cataract surgery and want to be independent from glasses. Others would answer with providing a multi-specialty experience that has the capacity to manage a large volume and wide array of ocular diseases. Another set of responses would be to serve the local community for their general refractive and ocular needs along with dispensing glasses and contact lenses. Each of these represent a different marketplace to consider when making business decisions. Once your resource is identified, we can move onto higher-level questions and analysis to begin the strategic process.

Appreciating Supply and Demand

Importance

The central fact in these exchanges consists of one side having access to a particular resource and another side willing to give up something of value in return for it. Certain variables in each situation make one case different from another. However, distinct patterns develop over time regardless of the conditions. Prosperous practitioners recognize these configurations through experience and effectively implement strategies that maximize their return on these interactions.

If given adequate notice and ability to change the setting in advance, these same individuals also create an environment to further improve the outcomes. A chess game is a great example. Novice players are caught up thinking about their current move at any given moment. Experts are contemplating multiple steps ahead for themselves and their opponents prior to moving. The key is to think as many moves forward to produce the most advantageous series of steps. Again, it is not unusual to recognize that many economic theories are similar to those strategies played out in games.

Keywords

Market economy: The economy created when many different firms and households interact for goods and services in a marketplace

Law of supply: The idea that as prices for a good increase then the quantity supplied increases

Law of demand: The idea that as prices for a good increase then the quantity demanded decreases

Equilibrium: The price at which supply equals demand

Surplus: A condition when the amount of a supply available is greater than its demand

Shortage: A condition when the amount of supply available is less than its demand

Monopolies: A situation when one seller can supply all the demand of a market at lower costs than all competitors

Oligopolies: A situation when a few sellers can supply all the demand of a market at lower costs than other competitors

Game theory: The study of human behavior when placed in strategic situations like games

Applications

The relationship between buyers and sellers in a marketplace creates a market economy. There are basic economic principles that govern their interaction. These are the law of supply and law of demand. The law of supply is directly proportional to price. As the price of the resource is increased, the amount supplied will be increased. This is the opposite for the law of demand. It has an inversely proportional relationship to price where demand for a resource decreases as the price is increased. These curves change as the market economy varies. However, their meaning, along with the intersection joining them (the equilibrium point), remain the same.

This relationship can be illustrated by using the market economy for cosmetic blepharoplasty, in which Teymoorian Eye Associates participates (Figure 5-1). There is an equilibrium at a price point of $5,000 where the supply for available surgery by doctors equals the demand for that procedure. If the price is increased, there will be a surplus of supply that would result in unused surgical capacity. If the price is decreased, there will be a shortage of supply that would result in longer wait times before patients can have surgery.

This situation assumes there are multiples buyers and sellers participating in this space. There are instances when this dynamic shifts to where there are only one or few on either or both sides. Consider an example when there is only one supplier for a particular type of treatment such as selective laser trabeculoplasty. Teymoorian Eye Associates is interested in having the technology in the office to provide that service for its patients. The laser price will be controlled by the one company selling it due to the protection from patent. That company has a monopoly on the supply. The result is that they can dictate the selling price because there is no other competitor

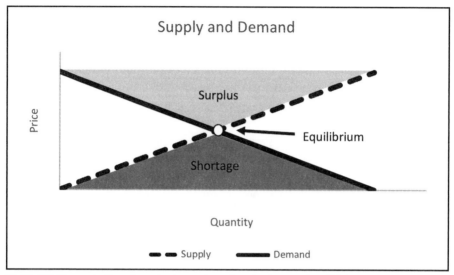

Figure 5-1. Demonstration of supply, demand, surplus, shortage, and equilibrium.

in that space. The company can adjust the price to create a surplus or shortage that meets their desire. Once new suppliers enter the marketplace as the patent for the laser expires, this creates an oligopoly. The dynamic improves for Teymoorian Eye Associates as prices will decrease because the original supplier will no longer have complete control of the availability for the resource. Similar interactions to these situations follow the principles of game theory.

Immediate Action Items

What is occurring in your specific competitive landscape based on the responses given earlier about the resources your practice provides? Remember, do not focus on all eye care but rather your niche in the marketplace. We need to understand the supply and demand in this economy. Who else is providing similar resources, and who is asking for your resource? This is the supply and demand, respectively, of your landscape. Where is the current equilibrium in this setting, and does it favor the supplier or demander?

In an ideal setting, your practice would be the only one offering the service in a marketplace that wants a lot of it. Unfortunately, most of us do not live in such perfect situations. Is there a similar marketplace that has high demand that you are not currently offering resources in, such as a managed care plan? Take time to assess the supply and demand in that environment. In the following sections, we will focus on building an understanding of whether those landscapes are worth entering for your practice. Remember, just because there is an opportunity does not translate into something worth pursuing. There are other factors to consider when deciding.

Minimizing Cost

Importance

A critical factor in this barter of resources is the cost of the good or service. The determined cost influences the resource price in the marketplace. The downstream consequences include the calculated equilibrium and other associated points. This drastically impacts the manner in which these interactions occur and eventually their outcomes. Top practitioners realize the complexity and importance of cost calculations. They use this knowledge to control the market environment and incorporate strategies that improve their results.

The cost is also a variable in the profit margin calculation for the resource. The importance of understanding the true cost is to allow evaluation on how to decrease it while still being able to provide it with the same quality. Careful use of this information enables continual examination of opportunities to reduce these costs. By thoughtfully understanding the definition of profit margin, a decrease in the resource cost is equal to an equivalent increase in the price sold for it. Smart practitioners attempt to improve margins by both reducing cost and increasing price. This approach optimizes business processes and permits the most efficient results from the resource exchange.

On the topic of determining cost, an easy mistake is to not associate all the costs that are involved in the process. This must be avoided to obtain an accurate determination of the real cost. The novice approach to calculating cost is to factor in all of the supplies needed to create a good. This process leads to one component of the overall cost. However, efficient businesses consider other factors that are not so obvious. An example of this includes the cost of the loss in potential income if the resources that had been allocated elsewhere. This exercise may reveal that another use would yield better results. It is this higher level of consideration that allows excellent businesses to separate themselves from mediocre ones.

Keywords

Fixed cost: A cost that does not vary regardless of the output quantity created

Variable cost: A cost that does vary depending on the output quantity created

Opportunity cost: A cost given up in the pursuit of creating an output

Sunk cost: A cost that has already occurred and cannot be recouped

Marginal cost: The extra cost when creating another unit of output

Total cost: The value of all costs incurred to create a given output

Applications

The following are types of costs that should be considered when attempting to calculate total cost: fixed, variable, opportunity, sunk, and marginal. Consider an example from Teymoorian Eye Associates to illustrate this topic. The practice is currently in a multi-year lease for one of its office locations for another 5 months. However, business is doing well and the patient volume has exceeded the capacity for this space. Another location nearby with a larger area is available to lease, but must be taken now. The current rent is $30,000 and would decrease to $28,000 since the new, larger location is in a less developed part of town. The cost of utilities varies but averages to $3,000 at the present location and would increase to $6,000 at the new location. The company just spent $4,000 in tenant improvements, also known as TI's, in their current location to paint the inside purple. There is an estimated $11,000 of extra income that is missed because of the current capacity problem that would be alleviated with the move. Moving expenses are estimated at $35,000. The penalty for breaking the lease is a one-time fee of $20,000. A decision must be made now to either stay in the current location or move to the new one.

Teymoorian Eye Associates calculates the cost of remaining at the current location. The lease per month would cost the company -$2,000 ($28,000 – $30,000). The utilities are variable costs but would save the business $3,000 ($6,000 – $3,000). The $4,000 used on painting is a sunk cost as it has already been spent and will not be recouped. Therefore, it has no value in this calculation. The lost capacity represents an opportunity cost that the company forgoes by not moving and totals -$11,000. There are no marginal costs. The total cost per month of not moving is -$10,000 (-$2,000 + $3,000 – $11,000). This would cost the business -$50,000 (-$10,000 × 5) since it has another 5 months on the lease. However, breaking the lease ($20,000) and moving ($35,000) would total $55,000, which would wipeout the cost of staying (-$50,000). Therefore, the company decides to stay in its location even though it is missing out on additional revenue because of its limited capacity.

Immediate Action Items

Have you ever looked at the costs your practice accumulates during 1 month or for each patient examination? It is easy in business to only consider how much revenue the organization brings in, but the more critical number is what is left behind after costs are removed. Is it worth working very hard to make $1,000 in revenue when your costs are $900 vs working less to generate $750 in revenue but only $500 in cost? You need to make sure that each incremental increase in the cost needed to create more revenue is worth the time and risk. As discussed before, just because there is an opportunity does not mean it is worth doing.

The idea is to work smarter and not harder. To achieve this higher level of business function, you need to understand your costs. Take time to look over this information for your practice with whoever helps in that area from your controller to revenue cycle manager. Specifically focus on things that change depending on the number of patients being seen. Then ask the question, "Would my costs increase or decrease if the number of patient examinations goes up or down?" Remember which direction would be most productive for you in terms of costs as this will influence your prices and decision making in the next sections. This analysis factors into decisions like assessing the feasibility of taking on a capitated plan.

Maximizing Price

Importance

One obvious discussion point when trading resources is the price. However, the determination of its number is complex. It goes beyond the actual cost of the resource to include internal and external factors relative to it.[1] A thoughtful understanding of these allows businesses to enhance the value of their own resource.

The internal influences are those that pertain to the product and its competition in the same marketplace. Resources do not exist by themselves. The price and availability of other products in the same space play a major role. Some of these will increase the selling price while others will decrease it. The goal is to create an environment that values the original product along with the other resources that complement it.

External factors also exist that influence the product's price. These include the characteristics and desires of those individuals purchasing it. It is important to understand the role that the products play in the consumers' lives and the degree to which they are willing to exchange for it. Successful businesses accept that there are variations on how consumers respond to price changes, so they select prices to optimize the return to the company. This ranges from sales that are low margin, high volume to those that are high margin, low volume. The important point is to correctly select the environment that better suits them.

Keywords

Complements: A relationship between 2 products where an increase in the price of one leads to increase in the demand for the other

Substitutes: A relationship between 2 products where an increase in the price of one leads to a decrease in the demand for the other

Elasticity: The degree of responsiveness

Price elasticity: The amount of responsiveness for a product supplied or demanded based on changes of the price

Price elastic: The condition where there is much change in the amount of a product demanded when there is change in the price

Price inelastic: The condition where there is no change in the amount of a product demanded when there is a change in the price

Applications

The determination of the price for a product would be simple if it existed in a vacuum. In reality, the presence of other products influences the price of the first. The manner in which they effect price depends on the products and their demands in the marketplace. When a patient has cataract surgery, the first service provided is the removal of the cataractous lens. The patient should not be left aphakic, so there is a demand for an intraocular lens. These 2 represent complements. If the patient selected multifocal lenses and is very happy with the uncorrected distance and near vision, the demand for glasses decreases. In this case, cataract surgery with placement of intraocular lens and glasses are substitutes.

Another concept to consider is how the change in price influences the amount supplied and demanded. This relates to elasticity. Consider a patient who just received her refraction and selected a frame from optical. The sticker price is $500. She presents the frame to the optician to get her interpupillary distance measured and continue on the purchasing process. The optician surprisingly notices that the sticker was mislabeled and politely informs the patient that the real cost is $750. The price elastic patient would not feel as strong for those frames and would look around for another option. However, the price inelastic patient would not be affected by the change in price and would want to proceed with the frame she picked.

Immediate Action Items

Is your practice pricing itself correctly in the given marketplace? This is where knowing exactly what you are offering is very important. Depending on what resource it is, the ability to change and set prices varies significantly. For those of you that are more in control of your prices, such as with advanced cataract surgery, have you benchmarked your practice to others providing the same supply? This does not mean that your numbers need to match the competition. To answer that question, you need to know your brand with regard to marketing. Branding will be discussed later in the book, but briefly, are you trying to be the low-cost leader with high volume? If so, you should be priced slightly lower than the competition with the hopes that the additional volume collected by more sales will outweigh the lower cheaper price. However, this means more volume and likely more costs to provide the service. On the other hand, are you providing an all-inclusive, state-of-the-art experience to cater to those with significant disposable income? If so, the lower volume of cases will need to be offset by higher-than-average prices. Your pricing and patient experience need to match your brand.

For those of you where there is less control over pricing, the analysis is different. In these cases, the prices are fixed such as those set by Medicare or capitated plans. The discussion about costs is even more paramount because the prices are established. Even though there is an opportunity to see more patients, can your practice generate enough net income based upon your costs. In the latter example, the cost to the practice may outweigh the gross revenue collected. This will depend on how efficiently your organization is operating. Based upon the pricing and costs, will this require our practice to see a high volume of patients? Is that sustainable and does that match your company's brand? Consider these points for your situation when evaluating whether you should enter, or even stay in, a given marketplace. Remember, you will not be able to fulfill your dreams of caring for patients if your company cannot stay open for business.

Optimizing Scale

Importance

The amount of a resource that a business should make available in the marketplace is another vital question that must be addressed. The answer to this is integrally linked to the cost and price. This analysis circles back to understanding what the company is, where it wants to be, and how it should be positioned in the market. These discussions help lead the organization to determine which pathway to take on such issues.

Flourishing businesses go through this exercise to carefully determine quantity production. They know the common belief, that making more product is better for the company, is incorrect. For example, there are cases when creating that additional unit of resource ends up having deleterious effects. It results in a negative profit margin. This includes problems with operations, marketing, financing, and beyond. It is in these decisions, which initially appear to simple ones, where their consequences end up having a large impact on the organization and influencing their ability to thrive.

Keywords

Break-even (BE) point: The evaluation to determine the sales volume needed to have the total costs equal the total revenue

Economies of scale: The condition where long-term costs decrease as output increases

Law of diminishing return: The concept where the value created for each additional unit output decreases over time

Diseconomies of scale: The condition where long-term costs increase as output increases

Merger: The business process where 2 companies join together

Acquisition: The business process where one company takes over another one

Mergers and acquisitions (M&A): The commonly used phrase to encompass the activities involving mergers and acquisitions

Applications

One frequent calculation that provides great insight during the decision-making process is break-even (BE) point. This analysis helps practices understand how much of a given product must be sold before making a profit. What is frequently missed is that there can be more than one BE point. They can reach a time when an additional unit of sale becomes more costly and outweighs the price (Figure 5-2).

The example of a pending decision at Teymoorian Eye Associates demonstrates this principle. There is additional room available to have another provider see patients in the office. Coincidentally, patient demand for eye care is also increasing. The company is evaluating the opportunity to add another associate physician to manage this extra need. The first issue is whether there will be enough extra revenue

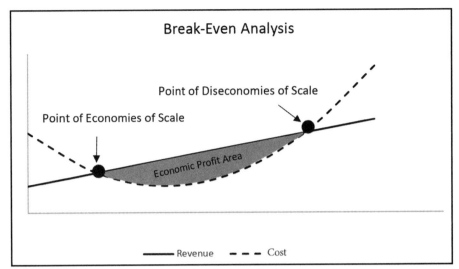

Figure 5-2. Graphical representation of a break-even analysis.

generated by the additional doctor to cover the new costs. These costs include the provider's salary and additional technical staff. The rest of the costs are minimal given the office size. The determination of the BE point would be at the junction of the extra costs and additional revenue. There is an economic profit after that point because revenue outweighs costs. This occurs because processes become more efficient over time with economies of scale.

An important note to consider is that this pattern of economic profit does not continue to infinity. There is a limit to how many more exams can be performed. This results in another BE point, but why would there be a second BE point? Once resources reach their limits, costs begin to increase as inefficiencies grow. For example, the extra patients scheduled to be seen result in more visual fields that need to be performed. However, there are no additional time slots available. Those extra fields are then completed after routine business hours, but they are now performed at overtime rates for the technician. That extra unit of work produces a decreasing return known as the *law of diminishing return*. It is like the first bite of a hamburger, which is great. However, every additional bite afterward does not taste as good as the prior one. These limitations eventually create diseconomies of scale. Beyond this point, the company is working harder and losing money. Also, employees feel overworked, and this degrades the company culture. Successful practices realize and appreciate these factors. They optimize their process and volume to maximize the return on the work they perform. Similar scale considerations factor into decisions such as mergers and acquisitions (M&A) on a grander level between organizations.

Immediate Action Items

Has your practice considered opportunities for growth to help decrease overall costs that would otherwise remain consistent? Earlier we discussed reviewing all the costs that go into your business to evaluate which could be reduced to create more profit. A subset of those costs was not modifiable based on your current company structure. An example could have been the amount spent on staff for the call center. There is no way to decrease it because someone needs to answer the phones.

During the analysis, you noticed that the process was not at capacity—the staff could handle more calls if needed. How can this valuable, unused resource be better utilized? This exemplifies areas where M&A can help decrease the cost via economies of scale. If your practice acquired a solo or small practice, the incremental calls to your center would not necessitate more staff. Your larger group can cut the cost the acquired group had paid. Certainly, many other factors are involved when contemplating expansion with other practitioners such as culture and brand, but opportunities can present to help financially that would otherwise not exist. On the flip side, caution should be given because the opposite effect (diseconomies of scale) can increase the costs. Getting big and working more can at times lead to less profitable work.

CRITICAL ECONOMICS POINTERS

* Understanding how others will respond in decision-making situations is critical to determining and executing your own moves—think of it like a game playing itself out.

* The real cost of a good or service is more than just the money spent making or providing it.

* Efficient individuals always consider the opportunity costs in a decision when considering options because resources are scarce and could be spent in other ways.

* One of the most valuable resources, if not the most, is an individual's time.

* Do not press forward with a bad decision just because a sunk cost has been incurred.

* The ability to sell a very scarce resource creates power while demanding them generates weakness.

* Although you always want to have enough supply of a product to meet demand, remember there is a cost to having surplus as it reduces cash available for other uses.

* Look for opportunities to take advantage of economies of scale when such advantages exist, but do not simply assume that will just happen by making more product.
* It is important to understand how price elastic or inelastic your target audience is to your services as this will help set prices.
* Consider offering goods and services that complement your core products to enable cross-pollination as opposed to substitutes that will cannibalize them.

REFERENCES

1. Sowell T. *Basic Economics: A Common Sense Guide to the Economy.* New York, NY: Basic Books; 2014.
2. Hazlitt H. *Economics in One Lesson: The Shortest and Surest Way to Understand Basic Economics.* New York, NY: Three Rivers Press; 1988.

6

Sharpening Negotiations

When opportunity comes, it is too late to prepare.

— **John Wooden**

INTRODUCTION

Active negotiations occur every single day in any setting where 2 or more people interact with one another. Simply put, negotiation is the art of making a deal. The competency for a practitioner to efficiently negotiate an agreement, both within and outside of the practice, has a dramatic influence on the success of the organization. Examples can be seen throughout the eye care field ranging from discussing salaries with employees to prices of capital equipment with vendors.

The approach to negotiations, including its execution, is like other stepwise procedures like refraction and cataract surgery. The key is to be well-prepared with a clear plan and a set of goals. With a proper understanding of the primary issues that are organized into a prioritized list, the principles of negotiation can be applied to navigate through any deal. One critical piece to appreciate is that, in most deals, there are many more dimensions than just the financial compensation. The ability to recognize all the issues at play along with the value they each bring to all sides characterizes an effective negotiator.

This chapter presents and explains basic negotiation principles to provide a fundamental support structure to use in different situations that occur in eye care. It includes a systematic approach that allows the reader to prepare for a deal-making opportunity. The end of the discussion presents various useful strategies to incorporate when working with different types and personalities of counterpart negotiators.

Teymoorian S. *Essential Business Fundamentals for the Successful Eye Care Practice* (pp 85-98).
© 2019 SLACK Incorporated.

The goal of the chapter is to train the eye care practitioner to successfully execute discussions that create strategic advantages. These favored results allow the practice to differentiate themselves from their competitors and develop the practitioner into an ideal negotiator.

WHAT ARE NEGOTIATIONS?

Businesses behave like individuals in many ways. One of the most common characteristics they share is that each has its own set of wishes and goals. In an attempt to realize these desires, agreements with another party need to occur. This process of working with another person or organization requires a series of discussions where wishes are traded back and forth between the sides. The purpose is to reach a satisfactory resolution where both parties are better for having negotiated together.

Effective negotiations do not happen by just having the two sides sit down to talk. The best discussions utilize a mix of art and science. Key issues are identified, positions on each are determined, and a set of breaking-point demands are delineated through the use of guidelines and strategies. Constructive negotiations generally begin with the countering sides having clear positions and insight about the items to be discussed. This requires careful thinking and analysis before meetings are ever held. Therefore, the single most important factor to have an effective negotiation is preparation.

Once the background homework is complete, the two sides can engage productively in discussions. The focus shifts from preparation to strategic collaboration. However, not all interactions in a negotiation setting occur with the counterparts behaving in an advantageous manner to get the best results overall. The influential negotiator understands that each interaction is different, both in issues and people. It is in this and similar settings when having a skill set to help the other side arrive at a more productive state is extremely beneficial. Despite all this time and effort taken to reach an agreement, sometimes the best solution is to know when to walk away without a deal.

NEGOTIATIONS IN EYE CARE

The significance of possessing strong negotiation tactics in an eye care practice is exemplified by the constant use of them in everyday interactions. Whenever there are 2 or more sides discussing a situation that needs to be resolved, the process of negotiating occurs. This is unavoidable as each has its own set of interests it wants to meet.[1] The successful practice owner accepts these activities' inevitable challenges and acquires the necessary competence to excel in those opportunities. This point stresses the critical importance of being prepared.[2] For those that are hesitant to partake in negotiations, they typically find themselves on the short end of these discussions that will occur regardless of whether they want to take part. The essential competencies in negotiations for the productive eye care practitioner to perform are the following: prioritizing preparation, considering issues and interests, establishing target and reservation points, strengthening alternatives, and applying negotiation skills.

Prioritizing Preparation

Importance

There are some individuals that believe they thrive in difficult times when the pressure is highest. They even use this excuse to procrastinate until the last moment to complete a task to induce the stress. However, most people do not share that same feeling as stressful situations do not result in the best effort for them. This latter group of individuals places value on the process of preparation. They feel most comfortable once they have had time to review, practice, and reassess their work. Otherwise, they feel their efforts will be incomplete and suboptimal.

Proper preparation makes every individual, including those that like to procrastinate, better during negotiations. Prosperous individuals understand that the process of getting ready allows them to complete their homework, or due diligence, on the relevant issues. This includes thorough research and thoughtful strategic planning before the initiation of any discussions.

Another important benefit to preparation is the minimization of emotional influence on the actual talks. A common pitfall of human nature is to allow feelings to affect our thought processes in the heat of a discussion.[3] This effect escalates with increasing importance of negotiations. Emotions can overtake the mind, which emphasizes the need for preparation. Readiness encourages actions and behaviors that are logical through strategic thinking. This approach maximizes outcomes while simultaneously preventing knee-jerk reactions. The value is the avoidance of questionable decisions when they are reviewed in retrospect.

This discussion does not mean that for each negotiation there should be an exhaustive preparation process. In reality, the amount of time given to get ready may be limited. The answer on how to best prepare in a short period of time is by practicing the process of negotiations beforehand.[1] Allow this activity to become second nature because of its importance and frequency in life. Preparation time decreases and its quality increases as individuals practice and engage in negotiations. This process develops skillful negotiators that produce high-quality results with the use of efficient time management.

Keywords

Negotiations: The art of deal-making

Negotiation grid: A preparatory guide created to identify and develop key topics that enables the use of thoughtful tactics to strategically maximize results in a negotiation

Milestones: The long-term goals attempted to be accomplished with the aid of negotiations

Teymoorian Eye Associates			
Negotiation Grid			
Situation:			
Parties:			
Stakeholders:			
Issues:	Interests:	Targets:	Reservation Points:
1.			
2.			
3.			
Priority Order of Issues:			
ATNA:			
BATNA:			

Figure 6-1. Template of a negotiation grid.

Applications

Most negotiations occur without much thought or fanfare because they lack importance. The repetitive nature equates it to that of driving a car. It is so deeply ingrained that, unless there is a dangerous problem such as an unexpected obstacle on the road, the usual motions are run through and a negotiated agreement is reached. However, when faced with difficult negotiations or an unusual driving situation, the moment of active negotiations is not the optimal time to think strategically about a solution. Chances are good that the individual will still be able to get through the discussion or past the obstacle, but the results are more likely to be suboptimal. This situation illustrates the old sports adage, "You play the way you practice."

The time spent on educating oneself about the mechanics of negotiating and strategies to achieve maximum results is invaluable. It begins by taking a systemic approach to understanding the scenario and utilizing a method that provides comprehensive preparation. This process can be achieved by incorporating a negotiations grid to prepare for and play out a comparable situation (Figure 6-1). These guides break down the problem into various key elements that build up to an effective course of action to incorporate during discussions. The goal of all this effort and time is to position oneself with a greater likelihood of reaching the desired milestones.[1]

Immediate Action Items

Have you ever formally prepared for a business-related negotiation? The time to do this is now when it can be practiced, evaluated, and improved without the costs of error. This chapter will revolve around an example of how to hire a new physician to the practice. Take a moment to identify some issue in your organization that will likely need a round of negotiation. Then, create a negotiation grid for it and complete it as we progress through the different sections. The following are some cases you can pick from if you cannot think of any to use: purchasing a new optical coherence tomography machine from a vendor, discussing your new lease extension with the landlord, and negotiating capitation rates from a payor. Now, obtain as much background information you can gather about the situation to best complete this preparation.

Considering Issues and Interests

Importance

Although negotiations focus on particular topics, what individuals think they are discussing in the same meeting may be different on each side. Part of productive meetings is the preparatory exercise of thoroughly identifying what are all the relevant points to be addressed. This requires each person to consider not only what is pertinent for him- or herself, but also what might be of value for the other side.

Even though one side may not consider a particular discussion point to be necessary, this does not mean it is worthless to the other side. Appreciating all the key issues opens up unforeseen opportunities that can further optimize results for everyone. The opposing parties place different relative values for the given topics. This asymmetry enables better solutions for both sides if each trades off what is less important for something that is of more value to them. Successful people utilize these comprehensive assessments that consider all the factors involved to create an advantage when positioning and executing during negotiations.

Keywords

Situation: The current problem(s) that need to be addressed in the negotiation

Parties: The different sides that are involved in the negotiations

Stakeholders: Represents the collection of individuals that has an interest in the outcome of the negotiation even if they are not physically present

Issues: The points of discussion that need to be addressed and agreed upon

Interests: The underlying reasons the various sides have each issue

Assumptions: The beliefs one holds about the other side and its issues

Applications

The preparatory process for a negotiation begins with the identification of why it is taking place. The purpose is defined as the situation. It is usually expressed in a statement using broad terms. This approach can be used to get ready for an upcoming negotiation at Teymoorian Eye Associates. The situation is that the practice is looking to hire a new associate to provide eye care.

Teymoorian Eye Associates has a scheduled meeting with a promising, perspective physician to fill that position. The parties involved in the negotiation are Dr. Snow, a physician partner at the practice, and Dr. Soto, the physician applying for the position. Although Dr. Snow and Dr. Soto will be the ones meeting, the stakeholders for this negotiation are larger groups of individuals. The following represent the primary stakeholders besides Dr. Snow and Dr. Soto: the other 3 partners at the practice (Dr. Teymoorian, Dr. Kim, and Dr. Raoof), and the wife and young daughter of Dr. Soto (Olivia and Emily, respectively).

Discussions leading up to this meeting have revealed 3 issues that need to be resolved. They are the starting salary and bonus structure, the number of vacation days in 1 year, and whether this position is considered partner track along with the number of years to reach it. The interests for the primary issues are different on each side. Dr. Snow and the practice are looking to hire a smart and hard-working doctor that fits the culture of the organization. This includes being willing to sacrifice short-term salary structure to eventually become a partner. Dr. Soto would like to join a large, multi-specialty practice that permits him easy access to ocular subspecialists and live near Olivia's family. He is not sure if he ever wants to take on the responsibility of being a partner.

Each side makes assumptions about the other, even if these thoughts are based on facts or not. Dr. Snow thinks that Dr. Soto will behave like a "typical millennial" and wants the highest salary possible while asking for the most amount of time off. Dr. Soto believes that Dr. Snow will think like an "old-timer" and looks for cheap labor to work hard and never offer partnership. Both Dr. Snow and Dr. Soto have these assumptions because of past experiences and what they have heard.

Immediate Action Items

Who are all the parties in your practice negotiation and what do they really want to accomplish with these talks? Take time to consider everyone involved on your side of the discussion, including those who are not present but will be affected by it. Although you will not know all of the details, answer the same questions for the opposing side from the information you gathered.

Establishing Target and Reservation Points

Importance

The point of having negotiations is to engage in an exchange process that results in the individual sides achieving their desired goals. Again, the value of preparation continues to this section on what the different parties wish to obtain during the discussion. Thoughtfully determining specific targets for each issue can dramatically alter the course of the negotiations and subsequently determine the level of success felt from the parties by the results achieved.

The goal of the discussion is to reach an agreement when each side receives their best-case scenario. However, this ideal state is not the usual outcome as they appear to be on conflicted sides for similar issues. It is more commonplace for the 2 parties to get acceptable portions on each topic. The best negotiators understand what they are striving for in a negotiation. They also know, more importantly, at what point the result is unacceptable for every topic. This absolute minimal point is the deal-breaker point in a discussion.

The importance of carefully considering and establishing these reservation values for each issue is that it represents the moment when a negotiated agreement will no longer be of benefit to the individual. It is then in the person's best interest to walk away from the bargaining table. Without this critical exercise being done beforehand, emotions have a tendency to encourage individuals to agree to unfavorable points just for the sake of reaching a deal. In hindsight, this leaves them worse off than if they had not agreed.

The purpose of partaking in negotiation meetings is to be left in an improved situation afterward. Thriving practitioners do not allow emotions to force them into worse results. Instead, they use preparation and sound logic to know when to agree to disagree. Not all negotiations should end with agreements or else there will inevitably be cases of buyer's remorse when the dust settles.

Keywords

Target: The goal each side has for the issues

Reservation point: The absolute minimum that each side will accept on an issue that will allow for an agreed upon result

Priorities: The organized list of interests based on a decreasing order of importance

Applications

Both sides will have their own targets for each of the issues to be discussed. Based on the practice's interests, Dr. Snow targets the following: $160,000 per year salary with a bonus of 25% after $500,000 of net income; 10 vacation days per year; and a decision on partnership to occur after 2 years of employment, although not guaranteed to be offered. After many discussions with Olivia and Emily, Dr. Soto has the following targets: $220,000 per year salary leading to a bonus of 35% after $440,000; 20 days off per year; and decision about an offer for partnership after 3 years of working.

Dr. Snow and Dr. Soto each have deal-breaker, or reservation, points for these issues. Dr. Snow cannot offer more than $210,000 salary as there is another very well-qualified applicant that will take the job at that number. The policy of the company used for all other associates, including those that became partners, is to start with 15 days of vacation the first year but graduate up after that time. The company also requires a minimum of 2 years employment before an associate can become partner.

Dr. Soto and his family are looking to purchase a home right away. The lender is carefully reviewing their application and is in the underwriting process. It is important for him to show a high salary to obtain the mortgage amount he desires. He cannot accept a job with a starting salary of less than $190,000 per year. He has reviewed Emily's surfer competition schedule and will need a minimum of 15 days off to attend those events. Dr. Soto is not in a hurry to know about partnership. However, he would need a sense of it within the first 5 years to provide him some assurance to his family's long-term plan.

Although Dr. Snow and Dr. Soto have targets and reservation points, they have different priorities about what is most important. Dr. Snow and the practice are very picky about new partners and would like to have the most amount of time possible to make that decision. The group has also decided that if the right applicant presents, they would be willing to negotiate the number of days off to start. Dr. Soto prioritized the salary amount the most because of its relationship to getting a home. Family time to attend Emily's events is also important but can be adjusted if needed.

A critical point to understand in any negotiation is walking away if the opposing side will not meet the reservation point on an issue. This is why the exercise of determining reservation points are done. It is imperative that these points are well-thought and justified. The credibility of each side depends on remaining true that they will walk away if these go unmet. The negotiator must stick to them. If not, the opposing side will no longer value these critical points as genuine and will attempt to exploit them. For example, Dr. Soto outwardly demands 15 days off or else no agreement will be met. If during the negotiation he considers options with 10 days, Dr. Snow will not take seriously any other mention of reservation points. It becomes a slippery slope. Once a reservation point is not met, Dr. Soto needs to walk away because it violated one of his basic needs.

The negotiation process can also be an emotional rollercoaster. It is easy in the heat of the moment to compromise on issues. If an individual crosses the reservation point, the result may leave that side worse off than if they had not negotiated at it. This is an example of buyer's remorse. Not all negotiations should end in an agreement because there will be times a satisfactory solution does not exist. If a side gives in for the sake of making a deal, then they will experience the same fate. Remember that all the time spent is a sunk cost in economic terms. It will never be recouped, so it should not be accounted for in the decision-making process. Just because Dr. Soto has spent hours preparing and talking does not mean he should accept any offer.

Immediate Action Items

What are your most important objectives ranked in descending order, and to what extent must you have with each to make an agreement acceptable? Create a priority list of wishes. Determine what is an ideal amount to obtain for each desire. Then, calculate what is the bare minimum for every one of them. Now run this same exercise about the opposing side from your current knowledge. Put yourself in their shoes as best as you can.

Strengthening Alternatives

Importance

The fact that negotiations can sometimes end with no agreement adds to the complexity of the interaction between the parties. There are some compelling reasons to have a strong backup option just in case negotiations fall through without an agreement. Elite individuals always build up their alternative choices because it carries significant value both during and after the discussions.

The obvious reason to have a great second option is that the individual negotiating has another choice if an agreement is not reached. Certainly, everyone wants to still be well off. The strongest possible alternative choice provides that reassurance to the negotiator. The other purpose is that a negotiator is placed in a more powerful position at the bargaining table as their second choice becomes more substantial. Better alternative options allow the individual to set their target and reservation points higher during the discussion. This is because the person would not have to accept anything lower in value than that of the backup plan. An effective method to capitalize on possessing a strong alternative is to inform the other party that it exists. The other side will either have to agree to more favorable terms or will decide that there is not enough common ground to permit a deal. It is always in the best interest of the individual to have the strongest alternative choice that can be selected.

Important note: do not lie about your alternative if you share it. If it comes out during the negotiation or later on, it can permanently damage the relationship between the parties. It also creates an unfavorable culture of what is expected behavior. Great leaders do not lie. They securely take their position, even if it is a weak one in a negotiation, and remain on the moral high ground.[4]

Keywords

Alternative to a negotiated agreement (ATNA): The alternative a party has if a negotiated agreement does not occur

Best alternative to a negotiated agreement (BATNA): The best ATNA a party has in a negotiation

Applications

Each party is aware that sometimes agreements cannot be reached. They have different stakes when it comes to their alternative to a negotiated agreement (ATNA) and best ATNA (BATNA) to select from should the negotiation culminate in no deal. One of Dr. Snow's ATNAs is to simply hold off for now, keep the position vacant, and look for other possible talent. The BATNA is the other applicant the team is satisfied with, although not as much as Dr. Soto, that would be willing to accept the position. This BATNA provides Dr. Snow a strong negotiating hand because there is a good backup plan.

The situation is totally different for Dr. Soto. It is very important for him to get this position at Teymoorian Eye Associates because of the proximity to Olivia's family. If they decide to have another baby, the child care provided by the extended family would be invaluable. Unfortunately, there are no other open positions in the area. He still has an ATNA, but it also happens to be his BATNA since it is his only choice. His option is to remain unemployed until a position opens in that area. The takeaway is that an ATNA always exists; however, it could be a weak and undesirable option that is far from ideal.

This discussion about alternatives stresses the importance of having a strong BATNA.[1] It provides comfort to that side when going through the negotiating process and can also be used as a point of strength. The dynamic would change significantly if Dr. Snow tells Dr. Soto about the other applicant and what her needs are to take the position. It would give Dr. Snow all the power to negotiate the best deals on each issue. Along the same line, it would be devastating if the best alternative Dr. Soto can give Dr. Snow is that he will be unemployed if they do not reach an agreement. The conversation would also change drastically if Dr. Soto did have a great BATNA. If there was another opportunity in that area with an offer that provides compensation closer to his targets on the issues, the situation reverses to favor Dr. Soto in the negotiations.

Immediate Action Items

Do you have a backup plan in case the discussion does not work out? Imagine what would happen if this negotiation did not exist at all. List your options ranked from best to worst. Is there a way to improve your other choices? If so, proceed with actions that will strengthen them. Now evaluate the same questions for the other side. Are any of your offers better than the best alternative they will have at the time of the discussion? If not, are you willing to give in enough to be their best option? Carefully contemplate whether you would be better off not agreeing as opposing to forfeiting more to reach an agreement. There is no shame on not agreeing on a deal. And no, all the time spent on preparing and discussing should not make you push a bad hand in this deal—those are sunk costs. If so, it is time to politely exit the discussion and keep firm to your decision unless there is new information to consider.

Applying Negotiation Skills

Importance

The value of preparation is not limited to knowing information about the 2 sides; it also extends into the strategies used during the negotiations. Excellent negotiators take time beforehand to train themselves on how these discussions can run and the dynamic interactions that develop. This extends into understanding the basic principles and methods to position themselves to engage the opposing side to optimize their results.

The other side's perceptions also play a critical role. These beliefs are partly influenced by their behaviors and actions. There are particular strategies that can be invoked during the process that enhances the starting, and eventually ending, position on issues being deliberated. Effective preparation prior to the meeting can pay dividends in the end. Not only can it achieve more advantageous end positioning, but it can also reach these agreements in a more efficient manner. If these principles are not introduced early in the process, the rest of the negotiation time could be spent trying to just reach the beginning position if it were applied correctly at the right time.

The other important concept to consider and manage is the role and development of relationships between the parties. Although efforts are made to keep negotiation discussions and decision making to business only, the reality is that humans and their behavior become part of the equation in the process. Effective negotiations understand their effects and prepare to deal with them as the two sides meet. This means being ready to interact with people of all forms of negotiating experience and personality types. Understanding how to react to the responses and behaviors from the other side becomes a critical skill to possess to achieve maximum results.

Keywords

Expanding the pie: The procedure to identify and enlarge the benefits of all issues in a negotiation to create more value for each side based on their priorities

Log-rolling: The exchange of smaller agreements on certain issues to achieve a larger agreement based on each side's priorities

Anchoring: The process of achieving a desired result by strategically beginning at a more advantageous starting point

Framing: The action of positioning a thought or action in a particular way to associate it with a desired effect

Applications

Negotiations begin between Dr. Snow and Dr. Soto after the preparatory work is completed. A common mistake that most novice negotiations make is to put limits on what can be achieved in the process. They view each issue by itself as if it is in a vacuum and try to get the most out of that point. They perceive every issue like its own pie. They want as much of the pie as possible for themselves. Indirectly, this means the other side gets less.

The best negotiators do not view these issues like finite pies but rather look for opportunities to make the pies bigger in size by working together. This process is expanding the pie. If successfully completed, both sides will be better off. This is a result of each side having priorities among the issues. They benefit from an agreement where they get more of what is important to them. One method to execute this expansion is log-rolling. The strategy is to ask for more on one issue that is important in exchange to give up more on another issue that is not as critical. Sometimes, it is as simple as asking, "What is most important to you in this negotiation?"

In the example at Teymoorian Eye Associates, the differences in the priority list can be used as an advantage. Dr. Snow is most concerned on getting a longer period to evaluate Dr. Soto for partnership while Dr. Soto values the initial base salary. Initially, Dr. Snow offers $160,000 base salary and a 3-year evaluation period for partnership. Dr. Soto replies with $220,000 and 1 year, respectively. Both individuals attempt to anchor the base salary toward their target number with the hopes of landing in that area. At this point, Dr. Snow notifies Dr. Soto that they have another applicant and that $220,000 has passed the reservation point. If Dr. Soto pushes on $220,000, Dr. Snow will end the negotiation with no deal.

However, on the new information that Teymoorian Eye Associates has another applicant and this is the only viable opportunity for Dr. Soto, he loosens up on his demands.[5] He shares with Dr. Snow the importance of obtaining a high base salary to purchase a house. This is an exercise of framing an issue. Dr. Snow appreciates the information and expresses back that the length of evaluation time is important to him. This allows for log-rolling to occur. They agree to a base of $200,000 per year with an evaluation time of 5 years. Both get what is important to them while benefiting the other. Instead of fighting over the pie for each issue, they worked together to expand it so they both are better off.

They continue this method of negotiating with the other issues as Dr. Snow is impressed that Dr. Soto wants more time off to spend with family. Dr. Soto in return understands that he is getting a much better salary than most start at and accepts a lower bonus percentage. They agree to the following: a base salary of $200,000 with a bonus of 25% after $475,000; 17 days off the first year that escalates by 2 days for every year thereafter; and a review for partnership within the first 5 years. Both sides are happy as they benefitted most on issues that were important to them, and neither one violated a reservation point on any issue.

There will be times when negotiations do not go as smoothly. Although there are many different situations and options on how to proceed, a few are valuable approaches that are considered universal. The first is to recognize that both sides are attempting to solve problems during these discussions. Helping the other side figure out their issues is just as important as solving your own.[2] Remember, unless the opposing party reaches a solution, it will be impossible to agree on any deal. Your responsibility is not just your problems, but also the other side's issues. The strategy is first to identify what the sticking point is for them and then utilize approaches to help them. It can also help uncover more critical information such as the order of their priority list, reservation points, and BATNAs.[1] For example:

"Dr. Soto, we have both been working hard during these discussions. There seems to be something that is holding you back. Would it be appropriate for me to ask what that is? I might be able to come up with some solution that can still benefit us both. I would be happy to think outside the box with you."

Another point to remember is that the opposing side is human as well. Therefore, emotions can get in the way. The process of negotiating, especially with those that are less experienced, is that feelings interfere with logical thinking. If tensions are increasing, it is best to attempt methods to de-escalate them. This involves changing the perception of the discussion that appears to be confrontational to one person vs the other, to an atmosphere of 2 individuals working together to address a problem. The key is to diffuse the emotions and focus objectively on the issues.[5] Look for commonalities to develop bonds with the other person. Also, remember to be polite and respectful. This generally leads to better and faster results. The worst-case scenario is you are left on the moral high ground. Consider the following reaction:

"Dr. Soto, it is amazing that we spend so much time in medical school learning about diseases and now we are stuck facing these frustrating business issues. However, I hope that what we learned in school can still be applied here. I am wondering, if it is ok with you, that we take a multi-disciplinary approach to this problem. This is a process we are both more familiar with using. Please let me first state my understanding of your position to check for accuracy, and we can work forward from there. I am sure we can solve this problem together, just like we do for our patients."

Immediate Action Items

Besides the obvious main issues that exist, are there any others that should be discussed that do have some benefit to negotiate about? Revisit your initial list of issues and reassess if any more do exist. Be sure to list any that could be important to the opposing side even though you do not value it the same. These items play a critical role as they can serve as pivot points in the discussion. You would not mind giving in on those issues because of the personal relative lack of value; however, these may intrigue them to trade in something you find useful. This expands the pie and gives insight to their true priority list. This information can then be utilized to further log-roll on items, thus maximizing the negotiated results.

Do you get a sense that the other side wants to agree but is having a hard time figuring out an issue? For any negotiation to work, both sides must agree. Place yourself in their position. What problem are they having a tough time resolving? Their problem is now your problem. If you can help aid them to answer, then they can proceed with the negotiations. As the saying goes, "Help me, help you."

If possible, initiate a practice negotiation with another person that takes on the opposing role. Practice speaking and thinking through the process discussed in this chapter. The more you practice getting out the right words, the easier it becomes. Then, when real situations present, you can focus your energy on the critical issues and not the words or strategies behind them. Prepare, practice. Prepare, practice.

CRITICAL NEGOTIATIONS POINTERS

* Preparation and practice are the keys to excelling in negotiations—do your homework.
* Although people negotiate with each other, separate people from the issues being discussed.
* Critically determine your reservation points because you will need to stick to them.
* Identify your best alternative to an agreement and work to strengthen it.
* Attempt to uncover the other side's reservation points and alternatives to an agreement.
* Acknowledge that your order of priorities may not be the same for the other side.
* Look for ways to expand the pie and not just try to take more of the fixed pie that is given.
* Investigation into other issues besides money can provide value.
* Help find accepted solutions for the other side, which will indirectly benefit your own cause. Always consider the negotiation from the vantage point of the opposing side.
* It is ok to agree that you disagree; know when to walk away without a deal.

REFERENCES

1. Weiss J. *HBR Guide to Negotiating.* Boston, MA: Harvard Business Press; 2016.
2. Ury W. *Getting Past No.* New York, NY: Bantam Books; 1993.
3. Stone D, Patton B, Heen S. *Difficult Conversations.* New York, NY: Penguin Books; 1999.
4. Maxwell JC. *Winning With People.* Nashville, TN: Thomas Nelson, Incorporated; 2004.
5. Fisher R, Ury W. *Getting to Yes.* New York, NY: Penguin Books; 1991.

7

Enhancing Marketing

The aim of marketing is to know and understand the customer so well the product or service fits him and sells itself.

— **Peter Drucker**

INTRODUCTION

Marketing encompasses all the work involved from promoting to selling products and services to consumers. In the eye care profession, this definition is no different with our patients. By taking a holistic view of this subject, it reveals that marketing efforts are extensive. The application of it occurs throughout the entire patient care experience. It starts when the customer first becomes aware of the company by finding it through a search online. This continues past the moment the patient gets home from his or her appointment and receives an email to provide feedback about the experience.

Eye care providers take part in marketing all day without even knowing it. Their actions and behaviors exemplify the company, which is a form of marketing. Patients witness this firsthand when coming through the office. Consumers' thoughts and perceptions are strongly influenced by what they observe around them.[1] This patient care experience creates the brand, or identity, of the company. It is this brand creation that smart practitioners view as an opportunity to improve the practice by differentiating it from the competition. It takes time to develop but can be of incredible value.

The correct use of marketing can separate a thriving practice from a struggling one even if the quality and level of eye care is the same. An unclear and undisciplined approach can waste a lot of money and not provide the expected return on investment. This chapter explains the method of how to incorporate marketing to produce

Teymoorian S. *Essential Business Fundamentals for the Successful Eye Care Practice* (pp 99-114).
© 2019 SLACK Incorporated.

an advantage for a business. The first section focuses on understanding the practice and its environment. Attention transitions to discussions about how to plan and execute the marketing initiatives. This topic progresses to developing the practice's identity and promoting it to the desired audience. The targeted goal is to develop an efficient marketing philosophy that creates value to the practice for the present as well as the future.

What Is Marketing?

The first part of operating a successful business is possessing a useful good or service to sell to consumers. The other part is to effectively promote this product to the right target audience. The completion of these steps leads to the generation of revenue. Marketing fulfills the latter requirement. The ability to do it well can have a significant impact on the company's overall success.

There are a few common misconceptions about marketing. The first is that the amount of money spent on it is directly proportional to the level of return on its investment. The second is that everyone represents the targeted consumer. The reality is quite different. Successful marketing revolves around the ability to efficiently research, strategically plan, and mindfully execute an action strategy. It is through these activities that a valuable marketing blueprint can be created and followed to achieve optimal results.

Effective marketing strategies are built on a foundation of knowledge centered on the needs of the marketplace and the status of the competitive landscape. This information is then combined with the company's vision and mission to design the best possible product promotion. The resultant marketing plan will position the business to efficiently progress toward its goals, both financially and philosophically.

This expansive process funnels down to the very important exercise of specifically identifying the real target audience. An accurate understanding of this issue helps to direct the marketing strategy to create the correct brand identity.[1] The result is an effective game plan that is supported by judicious and intelligent use of company resources.

Marketing in Eye Care

The influential powers of marketing are witnessed in eye care by the various types of patient cliental that are drawn toward a practice for its products and services. The best businesses understand how to effectively promote their products. This process forces the organization to identify what they do best—known as their *core competencies*—and which customers represent their desired target audience. The result is avoiding a common pitfall of wasted resources where the consumer base is too large or undefined.[1] This knowledge directs valuable company resources to be allocated for maximized return on the invested cost and time. The important fundamentals in marketing for the eye care practitioner to execute are the following: understanding marketing basics, developing marketing plans, appreciating the 5 Ps, growing brands, utilizing the Internet, and using the physical office.

Understanding Marketing Basics

Importance

Excelling in marketing is dependent on understanding the fundamental terms and ideas used for it. Their meanings shape the discussions within an organization and among its competitors. They also guide companies with their marketing strategies that provide direction for the business as a whole along with its individual products and services.[2] Effectively using these keywords enables businesses to separate themselves from others. This skill set is magnified in crowded landscapes that have companies with similar products wrestling for market share.

Keywords

Marketing: The management process of promoting and selling products and services

Internal marketing: Marketing to those within an organization

External marketing: Marketing to those outside of an organization

Pull power: The ability of a marketing activity to draw consumers toward a company for its products and services

Public relations (PR) firms: Companies that manage the outward image of a company and its associated products and services

Word of mouth: A method of advertisement that spreads recommendations about a company and its associated products and services directly from one past consumer to a prospective one

Print advertising: The use of hardcopy materials to promote a company's products and services

Radio advertising: The use of radio to promote a company's products and services

Television advertising: The use of television to promote a company's products and services

Online advertising: The use of the Internet to promote a company's products and services

Cause-related event marketing· Company advertisement done at an event that promotes a cause

Community event marketing: Company advertisement done at an event held for the community, which is usually near the physical location of business

Applications

Marketing in an eye care practice can provide a strategic advantage if done correctly. First, identification of the specific audience target is required. This then leads to creating a thoughtful approach to promote the company's services and goods to that audience. Marketing efforts can be directed to both individuals inside and outside of the practice, which is known as *internal* and *external marketing*, respectively. The goals for these different classes vary on the needs of the organization. Internal marketing focuses on the staff and is applied as a method for employee retention. The more common meaning is related to external marketing by attempting to draw patients to the practice. The success of these initiatives is determined by its pull power. Public relations firms are outside vendors that aid businesses that are unfamiliar in this space with marketing strategies.

The traditional route of marketing in eye care was achieved by word-of-mouth advertisement. If patients were pleased with their experience, they would recommend the practice to their friends and family. Examples include patients advising their colleagues at work to visit a practice because they had great results from cataract surgery or because they love their new glasses. The cycle would then repeat itself until the services were no longer valued by the customers. This method is still an effective approach to acquiring more patients.

As technology has changed over time, the medium used for advertising also transformed. The evolution has included print, radio, television, and now online marketing. These approaches are each unique and offer a specific connection to different audiences. The demographics of the targeted audience dictates which medium would be best used for a given practice. The utilization of print with a newspaper and radio is effective in smaller towns. By contrast, larger cities tend to perform better with television and online methods.

Another advertising method involves marketing at heavily attended events. Cause-related event marketing include donating money on behalf of the practice for the local Glaucoma Awareness Dinner. In exchange, the company is publicly thanked at the beginning of the meal. An example of community event marketing incorporates the use of hats with the practice's logo on them that are distributed at the annual Laguna Hills Fair. The takeaway is that the selection of marketing events depends on the audience likely to attend these activities.

Immediate Action Items

In the past, you have probably invested in marketing for the practice, but do you know which have worked best? An organization's marketing budget can quickly add up when all of the options seem so enticing. However, some will do better than others. Of the marketing decisions made, have you ever performed an analysis to see which ones led to increased revenue? Part of this process is to see which ones perform well so you will know the ones to continue. This requires strategy to track which advertisements are working. One method is to assign each form of marketing a unique phone number or promotional code. When a prospective customer contacts the practice through any medium, such as phone call or online, it will allow tracking to evaluate the advertisement that led to the referral. Analytics can then be applied to assess the relative value of each marketing approach. This will be discussed later in the chapter. Start marketing effectively by checking to see if your system can monitor the source of referrals. If not, take the opportunity to install a system that does.

Developing Marketing Plans

Importance

A functional business requires consumers that are willing to pay money in exchange for its goods and services. The challenge is how to connect the people to the products. This is very similar to having an aspiration in life. Without a specific goal in mind, the steps taken to achieve them have no target in place. The result is usually wasted effort and ending somewhere that was not intended.

Efficient businesses take time to thoughtfully understand the specific set of customers they are targeting to attract. Although this seems like a common-sense approach to marketing at first, the reality is that most organizations are so eager to start marketing that they do not critically assess their intended audience at the beginning. The excitement to have their product or service available for sale makes them take action before knowing where they are going. The end result is a wide and vague target of potential buyers instead of having a clear and purposeful segment of customers they are trying to attract. The repercussions of such random actions include the development of unclear messaging, inability to differentiate, and blown resources.

Once the specific audience is delineated, the next step is to understand the competitive space where the company will work and develop a strategic plan on how to achieve the goals. The due diligence needed for this assessment is incredibly valuable to the endeavor's success. This information identifies both opportunities and threats that need to be acknowledged. All of these activities eventually lead to an efficient marketing plan that remains dynamic enough to weather through storms but still arrive at the target destination. The lack of planning likely leads to poor and frustrating results.

Keywords

Market research: A process to understand the market space based on historical evaluation along with present-day surveys

Market share: The percentage representation of a company's product or service penetrance in a given market

Market expansion: The process in which a company attempts to find new segments of consumers

Marketing plan: The collection of thoughts and processes used by a company to promote and sell its products and services

Creative process: A marketing approach to foster the development and execution of a thought or strategy for a product or service

Marketing strategy: A section of the marketing plan that delineates the process of how a company's advertising will be performed

Market segmentation strategy: The process of breaking down a market and its consumers into a smaller yet more homogenous group at which advertisement is directed

Target audience: The specific consumer base that a marketing campaign is attempting to convert over to become customers of a company

Demographics: The statistical information of a group, which is usually that of the target audience

Customer profile: The characteristics of a company's targeted customer

Applications

Successful development of a marketing plan beings with an education about the competitive landscape that the practice will be entering in to work. Market research achieves this goal through a variety of methods. The most common approach is to see who currently serves the customers in the desired space. This reveals information about the competition and their relative market share. Opportunities for market expansion can then be assessed from that knowledge. The subsequent task is to define the customers that utilize the competition, which will indirectly reveal data about the customers. The culmination of these exercises supplies the new practice valuable intelligence when planning out its marketing activities.

Promotion is the next phase of the marketing plan. This involves advertising the practice's services and products to the ideal patient population. Its development begins with the creative process that produces some strategic options on how to achieve these goals.[2] The best ideas are selected and integrated together to build the marketing strategy. This approach is further broken to smaller pieces that focuses even more specifically within that patient pool to establish the market segmentation strategy.

The most important step in this entire process becomes the identification of how the practice brings in customers as defined by its target audience. The group's selection is vital as it provides the customer profiles and demographics. This information influences the entire marketing efforts and will be used in the metrics to assess its effectiveness. The simple rule of marketing is as follows: a clear understanding of your target produces clear marketing, and a poor understanding creates poor marketing. Within this audience, the practice hopes to discover some champions for the practice. Their intense commitment to the business can be harnessed in specific ways to further help promotional efforts.

Immediate Action Items

Does your practice have a marketing plan that it uses as a guideline for where and how to spend the marketing budget, or do you pick and choose marketing opportunities as they present? Without a strategy of how each advertisement plays a role in the overall picture, you will have results that look cut-and-paste. This will lead to a poor return on investment for your marketing efforts. Now that you know what your practice identity is through its clear culture along with its vision and mission statement, take time to assess who your target audience is. Be as specific as possible and sure it matches what is offered by your practice. The resources you provide (supply) must fulfill the desires (demand) of the targeted customers to be competitive in that marketplace. The next step is investment into understanding the profile of these market segments so you can tailor the advertisements specifically to them.

Appreciating the 5 Ps

Importance

Businesses that attempt to create successful marketing plans are required to answer some specific questions along the way. The request for this information will be inevitable in the marketing process and should be anticipated. The best companies prepare for these topics and provide well-developed answers. Underperforming organizations just continue their ineffective habits of generating responses spontaneously without a focused goal.

This information can be obtained through a process involving the 5 Ps: product, price, placement, promotion, and people. Once these are in place and defined, the ease of developing a marketing plan increases. Thinking through the 5 Ps is another example of how preparation is critical to the success of business similar to other areas like negotiations.

Keywords

Awareness gap: The space between what consumers know about a company's products and services vs what is really offered

5 Ps: The 5 components of a marketing strategy (product, price, placement, promotion, people)

Product line: A group of associated products or services

Product portfolio: The collection of products and services provided by a company

Churn rate: The percentage of customers that stop buying a product or using a service from a company

Cross-promotion: The use of one product or service in a company's portfolio to introduce and promote another to a customer

First-to-market: The condition of being the first product or service to be offered for a certain category

Trademark: A legally registered word or symbol that represents a company or product

Copyright: The legal right of an owner over literature, artwork, or music

Patent: The legal right of an owner for a design

Applications

One challenge that businesses face is narrowing the awareness gap of its customers. The patients recognize the name "Teymoorian Eye Associates" but do not know what services the practice offers. Therefore, the primary duty of the advertisements is to deliver specific information to educate the customers.

The 5 Ps of a practice's marketing strategy provide the required details to properly disseminate the information through the marketing activities. The following questions need answers: what are the specific products, what are their prices, where should they be placed, what promotions should be used, and to whom are the products meant for? For example, Teymoorian Eye Associates offers femtosecond cataract surgery with placement of advanced intraocular lenses. It is priced at $3,500 for patients with visually significant cataracts who are looking to be less dependent on glasses. These patients select their doctors by using online search engines.

One particular product or service does not define an entire practice. For Teymoorian Eye Associates, the various types of the monofocal and advanced technology intraocular lens options represent the product line for intraocular lenses. The sum of the options for all lenses used in cataract surgery along with a complete list of the other services that can be rendered, including refractive and glaucoma surgery, represent the product portfolio for the company.

Benefits of a diverse product portfolio is mitigation of the churn rate. Unless the patient with prior cataract surgery now has another reason to return to the eye care practice, chances are he or she may not return. If the practice offers other products of interest, the patient will become a repeat customer. Examples of such cross-promotion include glaucoma care if the patient is a glaucoma suspect or an optical shop if the patient needs glasses.

There might be times when a practice provides a new service or product that is an innovation in the marketplace and takes a first-to-market position. It is important for the company to protect this new advancement through trademark, copyright, or patent. Otherwise, some benefit of being first in a space will be lost as it will be closely imitated by the competition without recourse.

Immediate Action Items

Has your practice defined its 5 Ps (product, price, placement, promotion, people)? If not, it is time to carefully consider them. This exercise will help convert your marketing plan, along with its budget, into a productive strategy. Make a list of them now. We will talk more about these as the chapter progresses.

Growing Brands

Importance

The most important perception of a business is that of the potential customers. They are the ones that will make the decision to purchase a product or service. Effective management of this viewpoint makes the difference between successful and failing companies. All the expenditures spent on marketing serve as a means to that end. Everything about a business that the customers experience creates the brand of the company. Marketing is simply the way in which an organization's brand is maintained.

The best companies understand how to maximize their brand valuation and use that as a competitive advantage. On the other end of the spectrum, failing and underperforming business may not even be aware that they have a brand. Effective brand management provides the customers with critical information they need to make the decision to make a purchase. The first is to easily define the identity of the company and its products. This includes supplying details about what and where the product fits into the customers' lives and needs. The second is the importance of the company and its products possessed. This generates the value that customers should place on the products.

Marketing strategies attempt to create the best image and highest value for the company and its associated products. Exceling businesses implement marketing plans that focus on this agenda. This points out, once again, the importance of correctly isolating the target audience. It is this group's perception that must be managed. The next common mistake, after the one about not having a defined customer set, is losing focus on that group. The result is a waste of money and resources through inefficient branding. The best companies are excellent at managing their brand. They constantly remember who they are trying to sell to when making marketing decisions.

Keywords

Brand identity: The unique characteristics of a product or service as created by the company

Brand recall: A measure of how well consumers relate a brand to its class of products

Brand equity: The value of a brand based on consumer perception as opposed to the actual goods and services

Customer perception: The feelings and thoughts consumers have for a company's brand and its category

Applications

Marketing strategies are implemented to help shape customer perceptions toward a particular goal set by the practice. The specific associations that companies wish to create vary from one to another. However, the objective is to align certain characteristics with what the practice is, or hopes to be, in regard to their position in the marketplace. This combination of traits defines the business and develops their brand identity. The brand identity is similar to a person's identity in that it tells others who they are as described through various characteristics.

The strength of a practice's brand identity will directly influence its brand recall. For example, if Teymoorian Eye Associates is well established in the community and known to provide excellent cataract surgery outcomes, patients will associate the practice when they encounter the subject of cataracts. However, there will not be a strong association with cataracts if the practice's identity is not well known. The goal is to develop a positive brand identity with a strong brand recall to the desired associations.

The combination of the company's brand identity and recall create a value among its targeted audience that is known as its *brand equity*. This is exemplified when comparing a branded glaucoma eye drop to a generic one. If the company that owns the branded medication has developed a positive brand identity and strong brand recall, their medicine will be valued high because of the brand equity. On the other hand, another business that owns a branded medicine that does not have the same identity or recall will have a lower equity. The trouble with little equity is that patients will not value it as much and are more likely to get the generic medication. The extra value a patient places on the branded medication will justify the additional expense. Their decision to pick between the branded and generic eye drop will depend on brand equity.

The amount of brand equity owned by an eye care practice is vital to how it is positioned in the competitive landscape. Elite businesses work diligently to develop and maintain high brand equity with the purpose to place themselves in the most advantageous position in the marketplace. This process includes the implementation of marketing activities to alert prospective patients to their brand identity and indirectly improve brand recall. If the marketing strategy is executed correctly, the net result is that the practice's brand equity will increase among the targeted audience.

Immediate Action Items

What is your practice's brand? In 1 to 2 sentences, succinctly define what you think is the brand. Ask the same questions from a diverse group of individuals at your practice ranging from the leadership team to all the way down to recent hires. Does their description synchronize with yours? If not, work with your staff to train them about what is the desired brand. This lets them know where you want the practice's image to go. Next, does the company's perception of its brand align with your targeted audience? One easy way is to look over your reviews online or those written out by patients. From their comments, you can determine if it matches. The further separated the desired and real brand are, the more work must be put in to rebranding your practice. This will help focus your marketing effects by either spending energy to develop the brand or working to maintain it. The marketing tactics differ based on these needs.

Utilizing the Internet

Importance

One similar trait among leading organizations is the ability to remain flexible and adapt to changes when their working landscape evolves. There is no bigger example than the Internet's rapid introduction and significant influence. It has changed many aspects of how customers are led to make their purchasing decisions. This provides the opportunistic organizations a chance to excel if they are properly equipped to engage in that space.

The natural connection of a customer between the Internet and a company is its website. Effective websites are vital to an organization's success. They serve a plethora of critical roles including marketing through education, operations via appointment management, and information technology by patient portals. This is further magnified as customers have more universal access to it. Examples of these are the rapid growth of tablets and smartphones along with Wi-Fi. A properly functioning and easily navigated website is more of an expected part of customer service and interface as opposed to just an added benefit.

The leading businesses also understand how to maximize traffic to and through their website. The Internet is not a physical place. Customers must search to find websites. This demonstrates the importance of possessing an easily located website. If customers cannot get to and use a company's website, it may as well not exist at all. Successful companies understand how their customers find them and then figure out ways to make this process as simple as possible. Nowadays, that is through the Internet and search engines, respectively. The critical activity for this topic is search engine optimization (SEO). Along with its associated list of website analytics, optimizing SEO should be an essential activity in any marketing strategy.

Keywords

Web identity: The summation of everything on the Internet that mentions and relates to a company along with its products and services

Customer ratings: The grading of a company's products and services

Domain name: A company's website address

Site map: A list of the different pages that a user can access on a website

Landing page: The page on a company's website where traffic from other sites is directed to start

Content: The information presented on a company's website

Buttons: A graphical interface on a website that creates an action when clicked

Calls to action: A method to increase leads on a website where interactivity between the viewer and website results in additional actions that is of interest to the viewer

Testimonials: Customer review statements about a company's products and services

Blog: An online form of writing about a topic in an informal manner

Vlog: A video blog

Opt-in: A method of consumer recruitment where the consumer elects to be included

Opt-out: A method of consumer recruitment where the consumer elects to be excluded

Search engine: A program that identifies appropriate sites from a database given the set of keywords entered

Search engine optimization (SEO): The methods used to improve the ranking of a website when a search engine is used

Pay-per-click (PPC) advertising: A method of online advertisement where every time a viewer clicks on a company's advisement, there is a charge to the company

Retargeting: A method of remarketing used online when a consumer that has visited a website is shown an advertisement of a company's product or service later on in the consumer's browsing

Banner ads: An advertisement placed on websites that are routinely seen at the top of the page

Website analytics: The process of obtaining, measuring, and analyzing data from the use of a website in order to improve its performance and positioning

Website traffic: The movement of users entering and leaving a website

Session users: The number of unique viewers of a website

Pages per session: The number of pages viewed by a user on a website

Bounce rate: A percentage used to describe the effectiveness of a website to keep the attention of the viewer, which is measured by the number of viewers that enter and leave the site quickly as opposed to those that stay and browse

View-through rate (VTR): The percentage of consumers that view a company's ad and visit the company's website soon after

Conversion rate: The percentage of viewers entering a website that will produce a desired result, such as purchasing a product or service

Hypertext markup language (HTML): A particular type of coding used in website design that does not change in layout despite a change in display

Responsive design: A design structure of a website and its layout to keep it flexible depending on the display used by the consumer

Social media: The various methods used for the purpose of social networking

Social networking: The use of social media to create and communicate content that is shared with others that are connected to the creator

Applications

Eye care practices striving to be successfully must understand the role the Internet plays for their company and how to maximize its applications to benefit the business. The centerpiece of the practice's marketing focuses on the Internet is its web identity. Similar to brand identity, the web identity for a business represents everything associated to it that can be found on the Internet. This includes the company's website, social media accounts, and online advertisements. All of these pieces of information combine to create its web identity. One of its goals is to improve and maintain the practice's customer ratings.

Current and prospective patients use the Internet to find the business. They enter or search for the practice domain name to arrive on the website's landing page. From there, the viewers employ the site map to explore the website's content by interfacing with it through the use of buttons. The website content includes all of the information the company wants to share with the viewer, which can include written, pictorial, and video representations. Additional features are calls to action, which provide further user engagements such as, "Click here to assess your risk for developing glaucoma." The website can also post patient testimonials about what others have experienced and their feedback about the practice and its services.

Another method of providing content are blogs that are written or vlogs that are videotaped by the doctors or staff. Examples include the practice's retina specialist discussing macular degeneration and new medications for use, such as intravitreal injections. Other features include customers requesting the practice's newsletter through the website. These can be educational pieces along with associated promotions and coupons for related products and services. The website can be designed for the viewer to either opt-in or opt-out of these offerings. The summation of these features provides the viewer the opportunity to better understand the brand identity. The downstream effect is to increase brand recall and, subsequently, brand equity.

The biggest challenge to every business on the Internet is how to let the targeted audience know that the company exists. This problem is circumvented by having users explore the Internet using search engines. They lead the viewers to specific websites depending on the key terms entered into the search box. The best practices will position themselves to show up first in the results. Being in the initial few results is important because viewers are more likely to visit these websites than those on the next result page. There is an entire discipline in marketing related to improving a company's position on the result page, and that is SEO. There are several strategies to enhance SEO. They range from the use and consistency of key words on the website, the content available for viewing, to paying the search engine for better placement on the result page in the form of pay-per-click advertisement. Other advertising approaches to increase website viewership include banner ads and retargeting strategies.

However, before a practice can invest into SEO, it needs to understand what is happening on its website. This is where website analytics plays a valuable role. Its analysis provides the practice with an idea about its website traffic, session users, pages per session, bounce rate, view-through rate, and conversion rate. This information can then be harnessed to apply SEO strategies to improve search engine result positioning. Another factor to consider is how the website is being displayed to the viewer. Recent advances in technology have shifted the use of the Internet from personal computers and laptops to smartphones and tablets. Practices need to understand the vehicle in which their targeted audience is displaying the website to select the right display structure from HTML to responsive design.

The growing trend now and into the future is the presence and use of social media. There are several different applications that can be utilized to achieve success in this arena. Similar to the other marketing tactics, the important point to remember is the target audience and its profile. The practice needs to decide if the use of social media, and its resultant social networking, is worth the efforts to attract the viewers that use it. If yes, there are additional marketing strategies to implement that enhance the conversion of social media exposure to an increase in patients visiting the office.

One cautious note needs to be mentioned regarding social media and its use in marketing. The content placed on these is a direct representation of the company and is permanently available to view, even if content is removed. Care must be taken to ensure that the material presented is consistent to the desired brand identity and the practice's culture. Just like in life, it takes a long time to build up a great reputation, but it is very easy to bring it down.

Immediate Action Items

Does your organization utilize website analytics? As the world continues to change with data being available on demand at all times, your practice's website will either be a strong tool that enables progress or a hinderance that impedes success. For those that may not have a website and plan to continue practicing for more than the next few years, it is time to invest in a functional website. If your future is much longer than that time frame, then you should be looking to optimize your website to enhance the practice. This begins by looking at how effectively the website is functioning. The basic metrics discussed in this section can be measured using tools found online. Take time to evaluate your performance and compare that to benchmarked numbers that are also available for comparison.

Attempt to understand why metrics are underperforming and develop a plan to improve them. Are viewers overwhelmed with the material on the site or do they have a hard time finding what they are looking for? Making subtle changes to better fit the needs of viewers will help with SEO. Once alterations are made, assess whether the changes were positive by revisiting your metrics. Sustained improvement is the goal, which does not happen overnight. Stay committed and work through the problem.

Using the Physical Office

Importance

The actual office location where a business functions retains value with regard to marketing despite the growing popularity of the Internet and its virtual space. In medicine, this provides an opportunity for organizations to capitalize on the fact that patients still need to physically spend time in the office. The best practices identify and maximize this opportunity to further promote themselves.

This approach emphasizes the importance of a well-developed marketing plan. Even within the office itself, there are different locations that serve unique purposes. These subdivisions can have different marketing strategies incorporated to best advance the needs of the organization. Successful companies think about the entire patient experience and tailor this process to match their marketing along the way. Otherwise, opportunities to promote the practice are missed that could have provided more cost-effective methods.

Keywords

Brick and mortar: A physical building for a company
Banners: An advertisement placed at the physical location of a company
Atmosphere: The feeling and image that is created in an office based on design and decorations

Applications

The brick and mortar used by the practice offers additional opportunity to execute tactics from the marketing strategy. This includes indoor and outdoor banners that advertise the company's name along with its products and services. The most relevant piece is the atmosphere of the office because the practice of eye care occurs there. The moment the patient approaches the building is when the company must validate everything that was advertised in its marketing. All of the marketing activities provide the "talk the talk" component, but it is the physical office itself that must "walk the walk." This includes the call center, which is generally the first point of patient-practice contact. The reward for successfully fulfilling the patient's expectations from what was advertised is trust. Once the practice delivers on its promises, regular patients become champions and the company grows its brand equity. It is imperative that all the sections of business discussed in this book align and work together to produce the best and consistent patient experience.

Immediate Action Items

Is your office ready to deliver on the promises made by the marketing effects? Although patients give feedback through many mediums, these can be biased based on many factors. One approach is to have a trustworthy friend or family member that is unfamiliar to your staff come in for an evaluation. Ask him or her to be honest about the experience. Specifically ask what was good so you can provide positive feedback to continue that behavior. For anything negative, take the criticism constructively and initiate change for improvement if substantiated.

Let us get back for a moment to online reviews. Be prepared because it is seldom that you do not find any negative ones. How do you deal with such reviews? Take a two-pronged approach. The first is how to raise the rating back up. Since you cannot get rid of bad comments, the best solution is to surround them with many good reviews. Encourage patients to give you feedback online. Although it may not feel this way, most patients are generally happy with their service, but we just tend to perseverate on the bad interactions. Never negatively respond back to a critical review. It can lead to a HIPAA violation and gives a bad look to the practice. At most, ask the patient to call you to discuss any problems in person.

The second is what to do with the criticism. It is natural to brush it off using an excuse of your choice, but ask yourself honestly: is what they said true? If you do not know the answer, then look at your practice to assess its validity. Successful individuals and their practice use any feedback to their advantage; it is just hard to do when the opinion is negative. Get over the hurt feelings and then use it to better run your business and care for patients.

Critical Marketing Pointers

* Identify your target audience first before thinking about any marketing.
* During the process of market planning, still do not forget the specific target audience.
* Have a clear understanding of what your brand and the company's goals are so that the types of marketing activities optimize your financial and time investment.
* Take measures to keep the content on your website streamlined and consistent in order to improve SEO.
* Create a website that meets the needs of those you are targeting to or those responsible for making those decisions.
* Look for marketing opportunities to cross-promote lines in your product portfolio.

* Tailor all of your advertisement methods, including social media, to align with your target audience.
* Developing brand equity takes time but in the long term can create value both with returning and new customers.
* A great reputation is difficult to build and easy to lose.
* Take time to set metrics in place that will enable you to make sound decisions about where to continue spending your marketing budget.

REFERENCES

1. Ries A, Trout J. *The 22 Immutable Laws of Marketing.* New York, NY: Harper Business; 1993.
2. Kamauff J. *Manager's Guide to Operations Management.* Madison, WI: The McGraw-Hill Companies, Incorporated; 2010.

8

Integrating Information Technology

The first rule of any technology used in a business is that automation applied to an efficient operation will magnify the efficiency. The second is that automation applied to an inefficient operation will magnify the inefficiency.

— Bill Gates

INTRODUCTION

The introduction of computers and subsequent development of information technology (IT) has revolutionized the lives of eye care providers. The center of all this innovation is data. IT deals with the way it is obtained, entered, stored, transmitted, and analyzed. Unlike other innovations, we are being required to implement these advances in the form of electronic health records (EHRs). Successful practitioners understand this unique situation and use these mandates to enhance their businesses as opposed to constantly fighting a losing battle against them.

The ubiquitous nature of IT can sometimes make us forget how much of it we use and rely on for our day-to-day activities. The most obvious application is with EHRs, but this goes beyond just documenting a patient's clinical exam. IT and its associated systems allow for the patient to be scheduled, insurance to be run, medication to be transmitted to a pharmacy, and the referral letter to be sent out. These stored data permit advanced uses including analytics that improve company processes, provide information that helps shape practice patterns, and report to health insurance and government agencies.

Teymoorian S. *Essential Business Fundamentals for the Successful Eye Care Practice* (pp 115-129).
© 2019 SLACK Incorporated.

The manner in which IT has entered our lives and its impact is modeled as a blueprint for how this section is arranged. The chapter begins with an introduction to computers and the surrounding technology that create the systems with which practitioners work. The focus then shifts to EHRs, which have revolutionized the process of how providers function. Particular topics addressed are the methods of selecting the tools and accessories needed, training other providers and staff on its use, identifying issues related to patient privacy, and optimizing the outputs provided by EHRs to excel in government-related mandates and payment structure. The goal is to take the investment the eye care provider has made on IT and return it manifold through efficiencies of systems in the company.

WHAT IS INFORMATION TECHNOLOGY?

For those of us belonging to the early Generation Y and older, we can remember a time when our lives did not revolve around the use of digital and electronic technology. Information was simply passed along from either word-of-mouth or in print form. The boundaries of our work and associated advancements in society were limited by the ability to locate, obtain, and transfer the needed data. This information was securely stored up and access was limited because of these barriers. Then we had a breakthrough—the introduction of computers and the Internet. The lost key to the lock on the treasure chest holding this desired data was found. We are only now appreciating the vast amount of data out there that are available and how we can use them.

However, this environment is not a static one. The technological world has significantly changed over the past 2 to 3 decades, and it will certainly continue to evolve rapidly into the future. This is primarily due to 2 main reasons. The first is the increase of access to this technology as computers in one form or another are becoming commonplace everywhere. Anyone at any time can tap into this information. The second is the rapid growth in the rate of this technological advancement. This is exemplified in Moore's law, which in paraphrase states this technology is doubling every 18 months.[1] The amount of computing power in our smartphones far exceed what was used for astronauts to land on the moon. The possibilities of our technology feel limitless.

How has the workplace changed given these parameters? What was once a privilege to have your own personal home computer to write a paper and print it out on a printer is already becoming antiquated. The desktop computer takes up too much space and we are trying to be more environmentally friendly by not using paper to print. Now, the better option is to utilize a mobile option like a laptop or smartphone and send the file using the Internet through email or posting it online.

This paradigm shift extends even further into the layout of a medical practice. Years ago, the perception of a doctor's office within a practice as a private space with a window view and large table. The reality is that all the room within a practice is a valuable resource that can be converted into more revenue-producing space to see patients. It can be more profitable to have physicians utilize a virtual office with mobile technology and free up that office space for other uses. The advances in IT changes not just how patients are examined, but also how physicians function in the workplace. The most important question will be whether we can harness and capitalize on the new possibilities this technology provides, or will it be an inefficient use of our time and money to incorporate into our daily activities.

INFORMATION TECHNOLOGY IN EYE CARE

The importance of IT in the eye care setting is witnessed by the massive amount of data about the organization and patients that need to be stored and processed to remain competitive in this landscape. The unique consideration about this situation is that there is an outside force, in the form of governmental requirements, which is necessitating the use of electronic data. Instead of allowing these regulations to solely have a detrimental effect, the forward-thinking provider uses this obstacle as a stepping stone to improve different aspects of the business on many levels. These opportunities range from the practice side including operation and finance to the actual patient care such as physician correspondences. The skill set related to IT for the top-tier eye care practitioner to perform are the following: comprehending IT basics, assessing EHR selection, optimizing EHR implementation, ensuring EHR privacy, and utilizing EHR for government regulations.

Comprehending Information Technology Basics

Importance

Change is inevitable, especially when it relates to technology. The introduction of computers and the Internet have dramatically changed our lives, both at home and work. Successful individuals accept that change will occur. They view it as an opportunity for growth and improvement as opposed to an obstacle. The key point to remember is that the technological world is evolving at a rapid pace. This stresses that not only should aspiring people take time to familiarize themselves with it, but also commit to its continual learning. In order to take advantage of this situation, there needs to be a solid foundation of IT basics.

Keywords

Information technology (IT): The discipline of how information is stored, used, and communicated through the use of computers as its most common vehicle

Hardware: The physical components of a computer and its systems such as a monitor

Software: The nonphysical components of a computer and its systems such as a computer program

Upgrades: The addition of new software or hardware to update the pre-existing ones

Add-on: The addition of extra software or devices to a company's core IT equipment to increase or improve its current system

Technical support: The service to help users with computer and associated systems issues

Interface: A method of connection that can take the form of devices or programs

Network: The resulting aggregate from a set of interconnected computers and their systems

Online: The status of being connected to another computer or network

Offline: The status of not being connected to another computer or network

Remote access: The ability to gain entry to a computer and its programs from a distant site or terminal

Website: The location of an entity on the Internet that connects to various associated pages

URL: A website's address

Virus: A type of computer malware that replicates and integrates into a computer and its system's programs and files

Malware: A malicious software such as a computer virus

Applications

The advancement of IT has been one the most influential factors leading to change in medicine. There is software available to facilitate the required work performed all throughout a practice. This includes registering a patient at the front desk, employing imaging technology to detect disease, storing the medical data in the electronic record, and billing the insurance for the provided services. A prerequisite to enable these applications is the availability of hardware. Examples of these are the computer work stations throughout the office and the capital equipment provided with the diagnostic testing.

The introduction of such advancements also brings upon continual change. These include installing the newest software for the company's optical coherence tomography and obtaining permission to use a feature to allow data transfer from the visual field machine to the electronic record. The addition of such upgrades and add-ons improve the current functionality of the systems with the hopes of increasing productivity.[1] One consequence to consider with this growth in IT integration is the need for technical support. Effective companies ensure that this support is readily accessible to their employees because its response time can have a significant impact on how the technology is perceived. Their help in troubleshooting permits the company to effectively use the technology.

The ability to interconnect all of these systems to work together using various interfaces through a network is valuable. An example would be the use of a laptop computer to interface between the physician and the electronic record, and then transmit that information through the network to arrive at the billing department for claims processing. This can be achieved by being online at the practice site or can be enabled with remote access such as at home. Certain applications can still work even if they are used offline.

A discussion about computers is not complete with the role of the Internet. The most common use of it for a practice is the company's website. It is found at a certain address using a Universal Resource Locator (URL). The information hosted on the site can be a tool for both patients and staff members. Caution needs to be exercised whenever the Internet is accessible due to the risk of being infected with a virus through malware. The consequences of these can be devastating for the practice by disabling electronic records, billing services, and company communications.

Immediate Action Items

How susceptible is your practice and its IT system to viruses and hacking? Unwarranted entry and damage to your IT infrastructure can create significant harm to patients, employees, and yourself. Do you have a company policy on how to mitigate this risk? If not, work with your IT staff or utilize information from online and your ophthalmic society to create one. Certain topics are common among practices: protecting passwords, encrypting sensitive files, and avoiding exposure from malicious email attachments. This effort works in unison with your compliance officer as they share similar concerns. Creating a secure IT environment is everyone's responsibility. One strategy to encourage IT security diligence is rewarding the staff at regular intervals that have gone without any issue.

Assessing Electronic Health Record Selection

Importance

The decision to introduce the use of computers and its capability into a business is critical because of its far-reaching effects throughout the organization. There are 2 major reasons why companies proceed with this transformation: it increases production efficiency or it is required from a governing body. For those industries where the latter cause is not applicable, the decision to institute computer-based technology is simply an analysis of whether the improvement in processes with the addition of IT will outweigh its cost.

This straightforward situation does not apply to medicine because the incorporation of EHR is essentially required. It is not absolutely required at this time since organization can elect to not use EHR but will do so with increasing amount of penalty over time. The unavoidable byproduct is the need for the capital that provides the EHR in the form of computer hardware and software.

The analysis for investing into IT is different in this situation. Therefore, the thought process needs to be revised. Successful organizations faced with this decision figure out and incorporate ways that ensure that the first reason is clearly met by maximizing IT-based efficiencies to their processes. This approach makes the requirement reason essentially negligible because it makes sense to embrace this change given its strategic advantages. In the field of medicine, the processes that need to be maximized all center on the wealth of patient data and its dissemination. The advantage to this large amount of information is that there can be many opportunities for improvement if the technology is properly implemented and employed.

Keywords

Electronic health record (EHR): A medical record that is in electronic form (synonymous with electronic medical record or EMR)

Data integration: The process where information from various sources are brought together

Electronic data interchange (EDI): The exchange of data between 2 computers or networks

Data migration: The process where information is moved from one source to another

Data archiving: The migration of data from one computer to either another computer or storage medium

Health information exchange (HIE): The secure and compatible sharing of health-related information between many different entities including clinics, hospitals, health organizations, and government bodies

Local hosting: The situation where the location of a company's server used for EHR is physically onsite

Remote hosting: The situation where the location of a company's server used for EHR is located elsewhere and made functional through the use of a secure software application

Applications

Eye care practices face the continuing demands for EHR integration into their processes. The change from paper to electronic charts is inevitable. Successful companies seize the opportunity to improve themselves in this transition. The ability to maximize this situation requires a comprehensive understanding of the external and internal forces acting on it, which include the government and the practice, respectively. Externally, the general goal is to improve patient care and access to medical services. Internally, the objective is to provide this care in a productive and cost-effective manner. The overlap between these 2 is the efficient processing of data.

The most important concept to remember is that this patient information being discussed goes beyond the medical exam. The reality is that the entire patient experience is involved in this process. There is data integration across the practice during an encounter. Obvious information includes the patients' demographics, insurance, and medical history. However, additional data are useful to be collected, such as how they decided to visit this specific practice, what are their expectations for a successful visit, and if they have other unmet needs they may want to pursue that the practice can also provide them. For example, the patient may also be interested in facial aesthetics or cosmetic surgery, which is possible because there is also an oculoplastic surgeon in the group practice. This enables cross-pollination in the company as the patient may have come in to get glasses and ends up also being treated for droopy eyelids.

This data processing occurs through electronic data interchange that permits data migration from one inputting source to another. For example, the scribe can access the patient's pharmacy information that was entered by the front office to send an electronic prescription. This process enables the data to be transferred over to other locations for storage through data archiving to be used later if needed. Once this information is processed internally, it can be shared outside the practice to achieve greater utilization and improvement in patient care through health information exchange. Successful companies find methods to improve their work while processing all these data. They align the EHR they choose and implement IT to maximize their own situation. On the other hand, suboptimal practices perform the minimum needed and view this as an obstacle. They fight it all the way and never realize its benefits.

All this information needs to be managed. This provides another area for the practice to customize its EHR to match its needs. Options to the company include local vs remote hosting. Certain practices may benefit from managing it onsite because they have the infrastructure and can achieve economies of scale. However, there are other situations where it may be in the company's best interest to have it managed elsewhere. This would avoid the presence of inefficient full-time equivalents.

Immediate Action Items

Has your practice made the conversion from paper to EHRs? If not, it is time to assess and strategize how and when this will occur. Given the current and future regulations, including growing penalties for nonadapters, this change is inevitable. List the major hurdles impeding your organization's change. Each situation is different, but this process needs to begin at some point. The common responses are cost, inconvenience, and uncertainty about which platform to select. These are real issues with accompanying consequences. The thought process of how to address this issue is to revert to your company's vision and mission: where and what do you want to be? Having a clear understanding of these will help decrease the risk and anxiety in converting to EHR.

Do not misinterpret me about this subject. The change from paper to electronic chart is both strategically and operationally difficult to execute. However, to take an advantageous position in the competitive landscape, it needs to occur. Here are methods to address the main concerns discussed previously: for cost, remember that salaries spent on employees to manage your paper chart will be transitioned over to IT infrastructure and support; for inconvenience, plan ahead and provide the necessary IT training and aid along with a go-live date that you stick to; and for platform uncertainty, survey what other groups in your similar situation are using along with those you may consider consolidating with one day.

Optimizing Electronic Health Record Implementation

Importance

The initial implementation of technology, along with its cyclic upgrades, represents one of the hardest challenges in any organization.[1] The shadow that it casts can be so large that it can become the greatest influence on the decision to even adopt it in the first place. The final factor to the success from IT additions depend heavily on how it was unveiled and released for use in a company. Forward-thinking individuals and business understand the delicate nature of IT implementation and the magnitude of effect it can create depending on how it is executed. They take special precaution at this stage. It should not be a surprise that those who do not treat these with care typically encounter disastrous results. The silver lining is that this is avoidable if done correctly. This stresses the importance of great leadership and strategies that align throughout the organization.[1]

The reasons why introduction of IT can be so difficult is that it both requires humans and changes to their long-standing patterns. Human nature, and its affinity for complacency in some individuals, needs to be a consideration for how IT is incorporated into a business and its processes. The positive note is that human behavior does eventually accept solutions that are easier. This result can be achieved under the right situation that includes providing the appropriate amount of support and education. The organizations that excel in this arena acknowledge this instinct and attitude. In response, they create the needed environment to facilitate this change.

The best method to counteract oppositional tendencies in human nature is to infuse positive human behavior into it. A significant proportion of the difficulty encountered with change is the uncomfortableness created from the unknown. Successful IT implementation, including EHR in the medical setting, can be reached with the strategic use of human resources. These properly trained individuals can lead by example and show others in the organization the new IT benefits. This supportive approach, along with the demonstration of how work can be improved, is enough to pass those high hurdles resisting change.[1]

Keywords

Superuser: An individual user that has restricted control to manage and administer a system

Trainer: A qualified user of a system that educates those using it

Computer-based training: The use of computers as a medium to provide educational material to users

Task list: A to-do list commonly seen in EHR where the creator of the list can be the individual user of the system or those connected to the user

Flagging: The act of highlighting data or a process to make it easily identifiable when needed such as in a review process

Electronic prescriptions (e-prescriptions or eRx): The act of using a computer system to prescribe medications for a patient from a doctor to a pharmacy

Electronic referrals (e-referrals): The act of using a computer system to create, submit, and obtain referrals from one party to another

Electronic faxing (e-faxing): The act of using a computer system to transmit faxes

Go-live: A specific point in time during the implementation process when actions performed on a practice computer program go to a real-life setting from that of a practice one

Applications

IT implementation methods across the practice can significantly influence the EHR's adaptability. A company can spend endless hours contemplating when to convert to electronic records and then which one to select once it is ready to proceed. The most important step determining success will be how it is incorporated and perceived throughout the organization. However, there is an incorrect assumption for practices not to overlook. They assume that the EHR will just be integrated into the daily employee function and current systems. The reality is that this requires resources in the form of education and time for proper training. Great companies understand that a particular EHR does not guarantee effective use. Instead, it is the human resource using it that makes the difference. Elite practices take it one step further by not only providing training at the time of implementation, but also continuing to support and enhance its uses into the future.[1]

Effective EHR implementation into a company follows a similar strategy of training with other disruptive innovations that are introduced. The first is to identity and enable superusers that have a mastery of the system to lead the initiative. These individuals need to remain current with the latest upgrades and add-ons. Therefore, they should be encouraged to attend user meetings held by the EHR vendor. They are the only ones allowed to make structural changes in the platform in order to prevent any unforeseen consequences that a novice would not recognize.

The practice then needs trainers that are responsible for educating the staff on how to use EHR. The trainer might be the same person as the superuser in a smaller practice. They are the only ones allowed to train others. The methods for education can vary but typically take a combined form using lectures and computer-based training. This includes demonstrating to the employees how to employ the system to increase productivity while decreasing effort. In-office communications can be enhanced with task lists, and analysis can be expedited with flagging capabilities. Additional examples of efficiencies include the utilization of electronic prescriptions, referrals, and faxing. Not only can these applications improve productivity, but they can also decrease the company's expenses. It also meets governmental requirements on the use of this technology. This illustrates the value of appropriate training during the implementation process. Once the proper education has occurred, the practice is then ready to go live with the EHR's use in real patient encounters.

The staff should be instructed to seek these individuals out when questions or issues arise. Only allowing trainers to educate avoids the propagation of incorrect training by preventing less knowledgeable employees from teaching each other. It is not uncommon to see the spread of incorrect or inefficient use of EHR capabilities when training occurs with those not adequately educated. For example, the practice may attempt to make a simple change or try to analyze data to only realize the manner in which the information was entered was a roundabout way that renders this request impossible. At that point, the company must incur massive and costly processes to clean up its EHR system.

It is imperative to have the proper technical support, especially through the implementation and go-live process. This is a difficult and troubling time for employees as they are experiencing a major change in their daily processes. Staff will view it favorably if their questions are answered in a timely manner, allowing them to experience the benefits provided from the technology. However, should the response be delayed, employees will consider it more of an obstacle because it slowed down their productivity. Their first impression can linger for a long time. It is easier to be productive with EHR if these feelings are grounded in a more favorable range.

Immediate Action Items

Do you have identified superusers and trainers for our EHR? It is important during any time of change to have supporters that are knowledgeable and willing to help. During the discussion of EHR conversion, identify those within the organization that will serve as superusers. Only these individuals should be given the authority to train everyone else. It is important to keep consistency with education because subtle unintended alternations may cause long-term inefficiencies and frustration. Create a list of who other individuals will be. Now make a commitment to promote continual training for them as well, including conferences and online meetings, since they will have the responsibility of making critical decisions. Give them the resources they need to succeed, and let them do their job. EHR conversion can also be emotionally taxing. Remember to thank them frequently as well.

Ensuring Electronic Health Record Privacy

Importance

The sensitive nature of involving medical information emphasizes the importance of security and privacy for the IT data used in EHR. The protection, and subsequent sharing of this information, should be high priority to the company. It is considered that way with the governmental regulating bodies. This aligns with the primary goal in medicine to best take care of our patients. On the business end, there are steep consequences for failure to comply with these regulations. This includes heavy fines for both the individuals involved and the practice itself.

Businesses have 2 duties in this scenario to be successful. The first is to understand and remain updated with the specific requirements for patient health information privacy. The ideal approach is to have one or a few individuals responsible for overseeing this task to remain compliant. The best companies value this duty and provide those individuals with the resources needed to remain current with the regulations. This can include training through accredited courses. These staff members must also be empowered to keep everyone else in compliance without receiving unwarranted personal backlash from them. Even though these tasks are vital, there are also unpopular to the staff because of their enforced nature.

The second challenge is to tailor EHR to serve its purposes in the organization for process maximization while abiding to the privacy rules. Whether use is for internal or external purposes, the data that are stored and transmitted need to remain secure and private. EHR provides methods that can improve workflow for employees and enhance the patient experience. Successful businesses find ways to create value from the money and time spent to integrate IT and EHR. The effort expended to these activities lead to strategic advantages that help differentiate the organization from its competition. Conversely, a lack of time dedicated to identifying and utilizing these benefits will not only result in a costly addition of EHR, but also harbor ill will with staff because no efficiencies were created.

Keywords

Personal health record (PHR): A copy of a patient's medical chart, in either electronic or physical form, that is held by the patient

Privacy: The condition of keeping secret or private (synonymous with *confidentiality*)

Compliance: The set of decisions made and actions performed to follow required rules and regulations

Health Insurance Portability and Accountability Act (HIPAA): The Federal law that restricts access to an individual's medical information

Patient portal: An electronic platform through which patients, healthcare providers, and their staff can communicate

Encryption: The process of safe-guarding sensitive data by converting them into code with the goal to prevent unauthorized access

Data sanitization: The process of converting data containing sensitive material to a safer form that can be distributed

Applications

Protecting the personal health record of patients is a priority for any medical practice. Patients have a right to privacy over their medical care and issues. As such, it is the duty of the practice and all those involved with the patient to maintain confidentiality. This is ensured through compliance in accordance to HIPAA guidelines. The consequences of not maintaining it can be significant. It not only can pose harm to the patient if private data are accessed or released, but also can result in substantial penalties for the practice. Therefore, everyone in the practice must understand how to and behave in a manner that maintains a high degree of security.

The conversion from paper to electronic records has changed the environment. This includes the subsequent protocols for how practices need to maintain tight control over these data. The underlying challenge with electronic records is the ease with which large amounts of patient data can be viewed, copied, and disseminated once an individual has access to the program. This becomes especially important as patients wish to have these electronic data accessible to them through the patient portal online.

Two types of infractions that commonly occur are instances when individuals either unintentionally or purposefully break privacy. Examples of the former include sending communications like emails or text messages through unsecure means that do not have the proper encryption. Another case would be sharing data like in research projects without first removing identifiable information through data sanitization. An example of intentional privacy breach occurs when a curious employee views a patient's record without a justified reason to access that information.

Excellent practices address these EHR privacy issues with a company culture that stresses the value of maintaining its principles. If the company's policies and behaviors align with its desired culture, employees will understand that it is expected of them to maintain privacy and will be held accountable to this duty. The following are examples: privacy training with HR when a new person is hired, continual education from the IT staff to all employees to maintain practices that meet expected standards, and unannounced inspections of everyone in the organization to ensure compliance.

An application of the last example is to have the Director of Operations walk through the office on a particular day and evaluate employee workflow to assess the security of patient information. They inspect that employees log off from their terminals when they are not in use. Also, they look for any sources when patient information can be compromised like personal data in plain sight of those that do not need access to them. The right time to take corrective action is during these practice settings before the company and the individual gets penalized for making mistakes during the real evaluation.

Immediate Action Items

Are your practice's email and communication methods secure and encrypted? Patient privacy in conjunction with HIPAA is a popular and serious topic now and will only come under more scrutiny in the future. The ease of use to communicate through different mediums, including email, make them attractive for busy practitioners. However, this information must be guarded safely given the nature of its content. Review with your IT staff the policies and procedures in place to ensure proper security for the various forms of communication. The most common is email.

Do your employees know when and how to use email that complies with HIPAA standards? Create a few test questions of clinical situation involving these issues and give your staff a pop quiz about them. Educate or reinforce as needed. Are there any other methods used besides email? Survey the employee to compose a list with methods such as texting or smartphone cameras. Review the options with IT and your compliance officer to ensure security. If they cannot meet the standards, then direct the staff to stop using them and provide alternate means that are secure.

Utilizing Electronic Health Record for Government Regulations

Importance

The adaptation of EHR in the medical field is forced in part due to mandated government regulations. Although some companies view EHR as burdensome, the task cannot be assumed to be complete by simply purchasing IT capital. The process of implementation must occur to satisfy this requirement. Businesses need to create goals within it to ensure that the assignments are being completed and reported.

However, this task completion is not the end of the project for the best organizations. They use the information that is generated, along with comprehensive knowledge about the regulatory rules, to create action plans throughout the company to maximize incentives from the governmental program. Similar to the employees responsible for compliance, certain individuals can lead the charge to address these challenges. This is another example of how efficient businesses transform resources spent to satisfy required mandates into opportunities that provide redemptive value. Otherwise, this simply generates more wasted resources without benefit.

Keywords

Centers for Medicare & Medicaid Services (CMS): The US federal agency that manages Medicare and also coordinates at the state level to provide Medicaid

Quality assurance: The ability to provide a certain level quality for a product or service

Meaningful use (MU): The process of using EHR to improve the quality of patient care where specific measures are taken to calculate metrics that are used to receive Medicare funds

Physician Quality Report System (PQRS): A method to report patient-care quality metrics to Medicare

Value-based payment modifier (VBM): A method to provide different payment to physicians based on the quality compared to the cost of that care

Medicare Access and CHIP Reauthorization Act (MACRA): A pay-for-performance government program to replace the current Medicare reimbursement schedule that is intended to focus on quality, value, and accountability through the use of a merit-based incentive payment system

Merit-Based Incentive Payment System (MIPS): A system derived from a collection of PQRS, VBM, and EHR based on MACRA

Applications

Eye care practices and their providers must work within the confines of the rules and regulations of those entities that have influence over them. Effective practices find strategic methods to function efficiently that allow their operations to be maximized. All this is done while remaining in compliance with the provided guidelines.[1]

In medicine, especially for those that treat elderly patients, this involves interacting with the governmental body of the Centers for Medicare & Medicaid Services. One of this entity's goals is to create a medical care environment that provides appropriate patient services to maintain quality assurance. The implementation of EHR is a result of this initiative. EHR is a vehicle to achieve meaningful use to ensure the desired care level. Information about performance metrics is extracted from EHR and reported through the Physician Quality Report System (PQRS). These data are analyzed and used to determine payment levels through an application of value-based payment modifier (VBM). The introduction of the Medicare Access and CHIP Reauthorization Act (MACRA), a governmental program that focuses on a pay-for-performance structure, incorporates PQRS, VBM, and EHR to derive the Merit-Based Incentive Payment System (MIPS).

The end result is that payments to providers will be significantly influenced by their use of EHR and the reporting that arises from it. Successful companies recognize this dependence and utilize EHR to encourage proper medical practices and effective reporting. For example, their EHR system signals to the user to enter required information and also reminds them of recommended practices. This includes alerting the provider to educate about smoking cessation. The combination of these methods ensures quality practices, which meets the goals of the governing body, practice, and patient.

Immediate Action Items

Does your EHR system have features in place to help the practitioners fulfill these regulatory measures? Perform a review with your IT staff to evaluate whether your practice is meeting the necessary standards. If yes, can the current procedure be modified to make it more efficient, such as modifying features in the EHR? If not, develop a plan to educate the staff. Review what these measures are and how that information needs to be obtained and completed to successfully address this issue. Like the prior case, determine if changes to the EHR system can aide in this process. For example, some are developed to not allow the practitioner to complete a patient encounter note unless certain data and actions are taken to satisfy these initiatives.

CRITICAL INFORMATION TECHNOLOGY POINTERS

* The actions and attitudes of the eye care provider about EHR and all things related, including HIPAA, resonate throughout the entire company—behave the way you expect your staff to do, or else you are setting up this process for it to either fail or linger around painfully.

* There is a cost to converting from paper to EHR; however, successful eye care providers can jump that hurdle, and they make it an opportunity to improve efficiencies all throughout their practice that ultimately do enhance patient care and the bottom line. Have EHR work for you.

* Early on in the implementation process of EHR, identify knowledgeable super-users and trainers to ensure that consistent methodology is followed by all users of EHR.

* Simple steps taken to understand and apply the tools provided by EHR can help significantly with government regulations and payment systems like MACRA/MIPS.

* As everything converts to electronic versions from testing to documentation, remember in each step to maintain patient confidentiality and HIPAA guidelines in your systems.

* Each organization needs to make the decision of whether they will manage their IT needs in-house or outsource them elsewhere, with both options having positives and negatives when converting to EHR.

* When deciding whether to perform an EHR-related task in-house or to outsource it, apply your knowledge from operations to develop efficient processes and economies of scale to make the right choice.
* Since it is impossible to anticipate and answer everything that can go wrong when you go live with your EHR, make sure to have the right support system in place to provide your staff with the resources it needs during this stressful time.
* It is every employee's responsibility to be proactive to avoid malware infecting a company's system.
* Businesses erroneously believe that the change from paper charts to electronic will cut costs by reducing staff in medical records when, in reality, there is a new cost of IT support to manage these virtual charts.

REFERENCES

1. Kamauff J. *Manager's Guide to Operations Management.* Madison, WI: The McGraw-Hill Companies, Incorporated; 2010.

9

Comprehending
Business Finance

Beware of little expenses;
a small leak will sink a great ship.

— Benjamin Franklin

INTRODUCTION

Most people first think of numbers and computations when asked about the discipline of finance. Although the association of finance to these is obvious, the understanding of their meaning is perceived to be far from simple. The addition of complex-appearing legal documents to these numerical values further adds to the intimidation. Business finance describes how a company manages its money through the use of various financial statements and their associated calculations.

Similar financial assessments are routinely performed by eye care providers at their offices and homes without realizing it. The only difference is that these calculations are done without using the formal names of the concepts seen in this field. For example, the development of new technology occurs at a rapid pace in our field of eye care. However, these advancements do not come free. Providers must routinely ask themselves if and when an additional piece of capital equipment will be worth the amount of money invested. In finance terms these questions are answered with return on investment (ROI), net present value (NPV), and break-even analysis.

This chapter establishes the groundwork for the principles, calculations, and standardized documents utilized in business finance. However, it focuses on the application of the financial statements as it relates to common situations an eye care provider encounters in practice. This is important as each of them provides a different vantage point when evaluating the status of a company. The goal is to enable

Teymoorian S. *Essential Business Fundamentals for the Successful Eye Care Practice* (pp 131-149).
© 2019 SLACK Incorporated.

the practitioner to feel comfortable when reviewing this information and using it in practical ways. More importantly, this section empowers the reader to know when things do not make sense to raise awareness for the need of correction.

WHAT IS BUSINESS FINANCE?

When most people are asked to word associate with the term *business*, one of the popular responses is "money." Certainly, the creation of wealth is a metric that is commonly used to assess the success of any business venue. Similar to how we need to evaluate the status of every different system in the human body to gauge its overall health, a proper understanding of how money is viewed though different lenses in a business is critical to evaluate its well-being.

The biggest hurdle in this endeavor is learning the basic terms, understanding the different financial statements, and evaluating the implications of these put together. Once these fundamental pieces are appreciated, the true assessment of a business can occur. This allows taking a complex entity and breaking it down to its simpler units. These smaller pieces can each present a unique view of the organization's money. In particular, this exercise explains the makeup of a business at a particular point in time, the degree of its success, and the way in which it transfers money over time. The result is an effective way to analyze each dimension of this complicated business unit to understand it as a whole.

However, limiting the application of this information to simply assessing the financial status of business would be shortchanging its value. This is the equivalent of someone taking another person's recipe and following it line by line every time to prepare the same meal. Why limit oneself to simply being a follower when there is an opportunity to be a leader? The successful business person takes that unique knowledge of how the pieces fit together and then effectively makes changes in the process to continually improve. The true goal should be to create an even better tasting meal. This chapter (and really, this whole book) gives you the ingredients and steps, but it will be up to you to make your own unique dish. In business, just as in life, it is this little bit of extra effort and willingness to try something different that separates the ordinary from the extraordinary.

BUSINESS FINANCE IN EYE CARE

The significance of business finance in the eye care practice is assumed to be the ability to comprehend the relative wealth of an organization. However, the application of business finance extends beyond this to the function of what the business is doing with its money. These advance topics and their utilization separates the successful organizations from the failing or even mediocre ones. Those with a firm understanding of their financial status capitalize on that information to make sound business decisions. The companies that either do not have these data, or even worse have no awareness to them, make critical choices about the future while being in a fog. At some point, this haphazard style of financial decision making will be costly. The essential skills in business finance for the eye care practitioner to exercise are the following: learning finance basics, appreciating the balance sheet statement, understanding the income statement, following the cash flow statement, and valuing money.

Learning Finance Basics

Importance

The financial component in any business is an integral part of it. There is no special exception for eye care practices. Businesses cannot operate without viable financial support, regardless of whatever good or service is being provided to the consumer. The common interface between an eye care practitioner and this area of the company are the traditional financial statements along with their associated computations. Every individual that aspires to obtain a better understanding of these statements, and eventually the finances overall, needs to learn the fundamental terms and ideas on which they are built.

Keywords

Business finance: The study of a company's management of money

Ledger: A company's collection of financial accounts

Controller: The individual responsible for a company's accounting (synonymous with *comptroller*)

Revenue cycle manager: The individual within a company that oversees the process (revenue cycle management or RCM) that tracks the payments from patients in a healthcare system from the moment of an encounter presentation until the balance is posted and paid

Generally accepted accounting principles (GAAP): A collection of accepted accounting rules and guidelines set forth by the Financial Accounting Standards Board

Financial Accounting Standards Board (FASB): An organized group of business professionals, including accountants, that provides the standards for financial accounting through the use of GAAP

Book value: The value of something as documented in the financial books of a company

Pro forma: A model of expected future performance based on historical data and projections that is formatted using the same guidelines as current financial statements

Stock: A representation of ownership in a corporation

Common stock: A rudimentary type of stock that offers its owners the lowest rights, including the receipt of dividends when offered or assets should the company be liquidated

Preferred stock: An advanced type of stock where owners are given special considerations during times of dividend distribution or asset allocation for cases of liquidation

Profitability ratios: A set of financial calculations that describes profitability based on financial markers

Return on investment (ROI): A calculation used to quantify the relationship between the creation of profits and payment of costs for an investment

Leverage: The use of credit from lenders to create profits

Debt-to-equity ratio: A representation of how much money a company owes in debt relative to the amount of investor equity

Debt: The condition of owing something to another person, business, or institute

Bad debt: A debt that is owed but cannot be recovered

Line of credit: A form of financing that behaves like a short-term loan from a bank to a company

Credit limit: The maximum amount of credit a company can utilize from a given financial agreement, like a line of credit

Principal: The amount of money borrowed in a loan that still needs to be repaid in addition to the accumulating interest after a payment is made

Amortization schedule: A schedule that shows the breakdown of a payment for a loan over its payback period that illustrates the amount of money that goes interest and principal

Applications

The strategic application of business finance is a fundamental characteristic of an elite eye care practitioner. This does not imply that the provider needs to extensively understand every aspect of a practice's financial statement. As a leader in the organization, the role of the practitioner is to maximize the skills of its employees, but also outsource for help when needed. This includes recruiting the assistance of qualified accountants. The reality is that the provider must know how to harness these talents to effectively use business finance as an advantage. The key is to be able to look over financial statements and identify where there are concerns. Some describe this as "passing the sniff test." Does it smell right?

The core of business finance involves the use of a company's ledger. These individual financial statements describe critical information about the practice. They are managed by select financial personnel in the practice such as the controller (also known as the *comptroller*) with a close interaction involving the revenue cycle manager. However, it should follow the generally accepted accounting principles (GAAP) set forth by the Financial Accounting Standards Board (FASB) to be useful and legally compliant documents.[1] It is important to note that the numbers in the financial statements represent the book value of the line item, which is also used for official, legal purposes. These documents can be formatted to be historical or pro forma. The smart practitioner does utilize the pro forma statements, but also understands that these are projections based on prior data. Care should be taken to comprehend how this information was calculated and what it means.

The successful provider is also familiar with a set of common topics encountered in this space. The first includes the use of stocks for ownership in a company. The issuance of stock is a method of raising funds for the organization. The type and number of stocks will vary from one setting to another depending on the company's needs. For example, an S corporation business structure will issue one type, or *common stock*. Other entities will offer different stock with special rights, known as *preferred stock*, in addition to common stocks.[1] The classes of stocks carry different meanings, such as in times of dividend distribution or company liquidation.

The next useful topic to familiarize oneself is the particular ratios used in business finance. The first is a series of profitability ratios that relate the ability to generate profit to a specific financial marker. These include return on assets, return on equity, return on sales, and gross margins. Each of these has a different meaning that signals to the reviewer the effectiveness of profit making.

Another common ratio is ROI. However, its calculation does not have a specific set of markers that are agreed upon for use in its analysis. It will change from business to business with the method they want to define. The takeaway is that ROI represents how successful the endeavor was at generating profit based on the investment needed to initiate it.

An additional important ratio is debt-to-equity. This number is important when lenders for a loan are evaluating the company as they look for situations where debt is low and equity is high, or a low valued debt-to-equity ratio. An adjunctive piece of information they also evaluate beyond the debt total is the amount of bad debt. This includes debt that cannot be recovered, such as owed payments from a buyer that has gone bankrupted.

The last general topic includes loans and the mechanics of how they operate. A loan is an advancement of cash or credit from the lender to the debtor. The debtor can use those funds now and in return pays back the lender the amount loaned along with interest. There are many types of loans. One specific example is a line of credit. This is a useful short-term loan where the practice can borrow up to a credit limit for use as needed. The benefit is that the unused portion does not accrue interest but remains accessible for utilization.

In the repayment process, the amount borrowed is called the *principal*. Successful repayment of the loan means that the principal was paid back. However, interest accrues as long as there is a remaining balance. Every payment from the debtor first goes to cover the interest that accumulated since the prior payment, and the rest of the amount goes to paying down the principal. An amortization schedule is used to describe how the payment is allocated to the interest and principal (Figure 9-1). The effect is that the amount paid to interest instead of principal is the highest at the beginning of the repayment process. A great approach to reducing principal quickly is to pay extra at the beginning beyond the minimum amount required. Generally, this additional payment can then be applied to the principal without being subject to interest.

Immediate Action Items

Do you understand your practice's finances? Start by identifying where its ledger is and who manages it such as your chief financial officer, controller, or accountant.

Figure 9-1. Example of an amortization schedule.

Amortization Schedule

Principal: $20,000.00 Payment Interval: Monthly

Interest Rate: 6.00% # of Payments: 12

Payment: $1,721.33

Schedule of Payments

Pmt #	Payment	Principal	Interest	Balance
1	$1,721.33	$1,621.33	$100.00	$18,378.67
2	$1,721.33	$1,629.44	$91.89	$16,749.23
3	$1,721.33	$1,637.58	$83.75	$15,111.65
4	$1,721.33	$1,645.77	$75.56	$13,465.88
5	$1,721.33	$1,654.00	$67.33	$11,811.88
6	$1,721.33	$1,662.27	$59.06	$10,149.61
7	$1,721.33	$1,670.58	$50.75	$8,479.03
8	$1,721.33	$1,678.93	$42.40	$6,800.10
9	$1,721.33	$1,687.33	$34.00	$5,112.77
10	$1,721.33	$1,695.77	$25.56	$3,417.00
11	$1,721.33	$1,704.25	$17.08	$1,712.75
12	$1,721.31	$1,712.75	$8.56	$0.00
Grand Total		$20,000.00	655.94	

Take time to review the accounts to get a sense of what comprises it. Although you will not understand everything, the first step begins by breaking the immense resistance to look at anything in the form of financial documents. Do not be overwhelmed. Take this task in small pieces. You will soon notice common trends and familiar principles based on the basic keywords already presented in the chapter. These documents will make more sense as you progress through the next section. Refer to your respective manager of the ledger with any additional questions to fill in the details. Not only will this provide the groundwork to grow your financial assessment skills, but it will also develop your relationship with those overseeing this critical aspect of your business. You successfully learned how the human eye works—you can do this!

Appreciating the Balance Sheet Statement

Importance

There are few official accounting statements that complement one another to provide businesses a look into their financial status.[2] Each assessment has its own purpose and value. The successful eye care practitioner has the appropriate training to knowledgeably review these documents, ask critical questions, and analyze the results to provide an understanding on the company's well-being. Each of these documents provides unique information; therefore, they must be used together to get the complete picture of the organization.

The balance statement illustrates what a business looks like financially at a specific moment in time. It can be split into 3 useful components that can be further broken down to provide more information. The reviewer of the document will see what the business has, owes, and is worth. Respectively, these are termed *assets*, *liabilities*, and *equity*.[1] Their relationship is expressed by the equation that assets equal the sum of liabilities and equity. This statement enables an efficient overview of what is occurring currently but also has the capabilities to provide much more detailed perspective in each of those vital areas. The result is a proper assessment of the organization's areas of strengths and weaknesses. Elite businesses add to that evaluation by creating goals for improvement and implementing plans for action.

Keywords

Balance sheet: A financial statement for a company that provides a detailed breakdown of how it is composed at one particular instant in time using assets, liabilities, and shareholders' equity

Asset: A valued resource owned by a company

Liability: An obligation that a company owes

Shareholders' equity: A representation of value held by an owner in a company that is determined by the sum of capital stock and retained earnings

Liquidity: A description of how easy an asset can be converted to cash

Current assets: A collection of assets that will routinely be converted to cash within the next year, including cash on hand, accounts receivable, inventory, and prepaid expenses

Cash: The most liquid form of money

Accounts receivable (AR): A collection of payments that are owed to the company

Inventory: The sum of all final products ready for sale along with any available raw materials

Prepaid expenses: The expenses that have been paid already but have not been used

Noncurrent assets: The set of assets that are not sold routinely and, therefore, are not converted to cash

Intangible assets: The set of assets owned by a company that have value but are not readily measured

Net fixed assets: The resultant of subtracting accumulated depreciation from the cost of fixed assets

Cost of fixed assets: The collection of property and equipment owned and used by the practice for its routine operations

Depreciation: A term used to express the decrease in value of an asset over time due to natural wear and tear from use

Accumulated depreciation: The total depreciation collected since the acquisition of an asset

Accounts payable (AP): A collection of bills or credits a company owes another party that needs to be paid

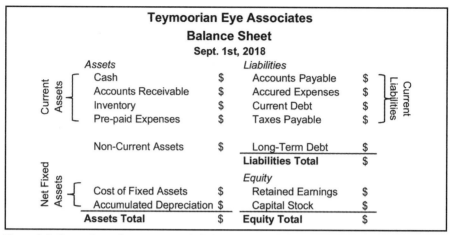

Figure 9-2. Categories and organization of a balance sheet.

Accrued expenses: The money a company owes for expenses it has accumulated over time

Current debt: The amount owed in loans that need to be repaid in less than 1 year

Taxes payable: The amount of income tax a practice owes the government

Long-term debt: The amount owed in loans that do not need to be paid within the year

Retained earnings: The amount of profits left behind that are not given as dividends to shareholders

Dividends: An amount of money paid by a company to its shareholders based upon profitability

Capital stock: The stock held by owners that represents the money needed to begin and add onto a business

Applications

The eye care practitioner utilizes the balance sheet to provide a sense of what the practice looks like from an outsider's point of view at a particular instance in time. Again, it is structured by the equation of assets equals liabilities plus shareholders' equity. The translation of this is the worth of the practice equals what it owes plus the owner's value. Just as in any algebraic equation, the 2 sides must remain balanced. Therefore, the addition of anything on the left side must correspond to a similar increase on the right side.

The categories of assets, liabilities, and shareholders' equity can be broken down to smaller components to provide greater detail about each section (Figure 9-2). The total assets is the sum of current assets, noncurrent assets, and net fixed assets. Each of these 3 can be further separated by subsections.

The current assets represent a group of resources that can be changed to actual cash on hand in less than a 1-year period. Its subsections are typically ordered in decreasing rates of liquidity, or how quickly they can be converted to cash. It should not be a surprise that the first group is cash. This includes all the money available to the practice such as in drawers and boxes. The next one is accounts receivable (AR). It denotes the money owed to the practice for goods and services already provided. The subsequent group is inventory, which encompasses all forms of inventory from raw materials and final products yet to be sold. The last one is prepaid expenses. This subsection covers all bills that have already been paid but not yet used.

The noncurrent assets section represents resources that cannot be converted to cash. The best way to think of this group is to consider all the intangibles belonging to the practice. This includes the name of the company and any unique operational processes that provides value. They are subsequently given a book value to show up in the balance sheet.

The last asset section is net fixed assets. It is the subtraction of accumulated depreciation from costs of fixed assets. Fixed assets are all the properties, equipment, and physical objects owned by the practice that are not meant to be sold. *Depreciation* is an accounting term used to discuss the loss of value secondary to natural usage. The process of depreciating an asset is a method to spread its cost over its useful lifetime. Consider the cost of purchasing a femtosecond laser of $500,000. After 2 years of use, it no longer has the same initial value. Depreciation is used to account for this wear-and-tear to provide an accurate value at that moment. Accumulated depreciation is simply the summation of all its prior depreciation.

On the other side of the balance sheet are the categories of liabilities and shareholders' equity. Liabilities are typically separated into subsections of current liabilities and long-term debt that illustrate what the practice owes. The subsections of current liabilities are accounts payable (AP), accrued expenses, current debt, and taxes payable. AP is the opposite principle of AR. It represents the amount of money the practice owes another business despite already possessing the product or using the service. Accrued expenses denote money owed such as salaries. Current debt encompasses loans owed by the practice that are due in less than 1 year. Taxes payable are the income taxes yet to be paid to the government. These items add up to the current liabilities. Note that loans that do not need to be repaid within the year are placed under their own section of long-term debt in order to keep these longer-termed obligations separate from the shorter, current liabilities.

The last category is the shareholders' equity, which is the sum of retained earnings and capital stock. Retained earnings represent the amount left after dividends for a company are paid from the profits. The capital stock encompasses all the capital associated with starting and adding on to it. Specific options include common and preferred stocks.[2]

Immediate Action Items

Have you ever looked at your company's balance statement? More importantly, was it looked at recently and is it up-to-date? This statement can provide a wealth of information about what is going in the practice; however, it needs to be correct to maintain its effectiveness. Start by reviewing the 3 main areas: assets, liabilities, and equity. Make sure assets equals liabilities plus equity. If not, you have a big problem and should question the validity of the whole document and the credibility of the maker. However, this also does not mean that if the numbers do match then it must be accurate. Follow your instincts; it should make sense.

Focus on what items are in each section to gain familiarity with it. Depending on the complexity of the business, the number of items can range from a few to many. Are the categories represented in clear arrangement one to another, or does it look jumbled? Even large statements should have a logical flow to them, just like words in a book. If not, ask the creator of the document to provide an explanation of each category along with an update. If that person struggles to give a basic presentation, then either the information is not effectively organized or the person is not comfortable with the material. Afterward, take time by yourself to look over each section carefully using the keywords provided earlier to understand their meanings. Continue to review the statement repetitively but add more detailed material with each look. This is just like looking at visual fields; it will be faster and easier with each additional evaluation.

Understanding the Income Statement

Importance

The income statement is the next important financial document to review. It provides insight to the overall health of the business in terms of its profitability.[1] The value of this statement is that it breaks down the key factors that lead up to the determination of whether a company generates wealth through its operations.

Businesses need to continually create profit to remain functional to create goods and provide services. The successful eye care practitioner realizes that to be able to care for patients, the office doors need to be open for business. This financial assessment provides insight on this area in particular. The best organizations use this information, along with the analysis from the other documents, to continually improve themselves. On the other end of the spectrum, those companies that do not pay attention to these will either eventually learn through costly mistakes or simply go out of business.

Keywords

Income statement: A financial statement for a company that describes and calculates its profitability through profits and losses (synonymous with *profit & loss statement*)

Income: The amount of revenue left over after all costs and expenses are accounted (synonymous with *profit, bottom line*, and *earnings*)

Cost: The amount of money needed to create a product that was sold

Expense: The amount of money spent to provide the ancillary support needed to create a product that was sold such as marketing, research, and administrative

Net sales: The amount that will be collected from a sale minus any discounts provided to the customer to entice the purchase (synonymous with *revenue* and *top line*)

Loss: The situation when costs and expenses exceed net sales

Cost of goods sold (COGS): The cumulative costs incurred by a company to directly create the products that are sold

Gross margin: The amount of money left over from a sale of a product after the COGS are subtracted (synonymous with *gross profits*)

Profit margin: A calculation determined by how much of the profit from a sale exceeds its costs

Sales, general, and administrative expenses (SG&A): A collective group of expenses incurred by a company to provide ancillary support that help generate sales. These expenses include sales & marketing, research & development, and general & administrative (synonymous with *operating expenses*)

Overhead: The cost that is incurred to make a good or provide a service that cannot be directly attributed to the material and labor for that good or service

Operations income: The income left over after accounting for all the costs and expenses from the net sales, which is represented by subtracting SG&A from the gross profits

Earnings before interest, taxes, depreciation, and amortization (EBITDA): A non-GAAP calculation used to assess the financial performance of a business to assess its earning potential

Private equity firms: Organizations that are backed by private, and not public, funding used to invest in business opportunities

Applications

The income statement works with the other financial documents to provide additional information about the practice. It is commonly referred to as *profit & loss* (P&L) *statement* (Figure 9-3). The knowledgeable eye care practitioner uses this statement to assess how the practice is doing by focusing on its profitability over a period of time. The document does not show whether the company actually has cash available, which is demonstrated by the cash flow statement, or what it is, which is described by the balance statement. The impact of these financial documents addressing different points can be illustrated with an example. A practice can be profitable on its income statement but not have cash available to pay bills or fulfill more orders based on its cash flow statements. The strategic provider understands the uniqueness and interplay among these documents to obtain a detailed understanding of what is actually occurring in the practice.

The general formula for the income statement is defined as income equals the amount of sales minus the costs and expenses needed to make those sales. The sales are sometimes referred to as *revenue* or *the top line* since it is placed at the top of the income statement. However, it should be noted that the sales described here actually represent the net sales. This means the price that was actually used in the transaction with the customer. The net sales accounts for discounts or reduction in the original sales price quoted to the buyer. The income statement then accounts for the associated costs and expenses. It eventually leads to the income. The income is also referred to as *earnings* or *the bottom line* since it is listed at the bottom of the statement. When the income is a positive number, it is a profit and referred to as "being in the black."

Figure 9-3. Categories and organization of an income statement.

Teymoorian Eye Associates

Income Statement (P&L)

Jan. 1st, 2018 to Dec. 31st, 2018

Net Sales		$
COGS		$
Gross Profit		$
SG&A		$
Interest Income		$
Income Taxes		$
Net Income		$

Operation Income

A negative number is a loss or "being in the red." In financial spreadsheets, the color black is additive while red is subtractive.

Commonly after the first line stating the net sales, the amount of money needed to make the goods that were sold are listed as the cost of goods sold (COGS). For example, this would represent the cost of the intraocular lens the practice paid to the manufacturer that was used in surgery. The difference between the net sales and the COGS produces the gross margin or profit. An additional metric that derives from these is the profit margin that expresses the gross margin relative to the net sales, or how much money was generated relative to the sale of a product after accounts for the COGS. An extreme illustration is the use of intravitreal injections. The sales of the injection are $3,000 but the COGS are $2,950. This yields a gross profit of $50 despite a sales price of $3,000. The profit margin is 1.6% ($50/$3,000). A mistake or inability to get paid for this injection would result in a large loss. Therefore, higher profit margins are better in general as they are more profitable but also buffer against unforeseen problems or risks that eat away at the margins.

The next line is a combination of all the expenses required to make the sales. It is generally listed as sales, general, and administrative (SG&A) expenses. Another name used for SG&A is *operating expenses*. It can be further broken up into smaller subsections of expenses depending on the company. These include sales and marketing, research and development, and general and administrative. Another term used for these is *overhead expenses*. It is not the cost of the item sold that is the COGS, but it represents everything else. The subtraction of SG&A from gross profits leads to the operations income.

The following section of the income statement addresses other considerations that influence the practice's profitability. This includes the income accumulated from interest that has grown from the cash the practice has in other accounts such as in banks. There is also a line for the income taxes that need to be paid by the practice to the government for the operations income. The addition of operations income to the interest income minus the income taxes leads to the net income. Again, the net income is also the bottom line, which represents how profitable the sales are after all other factors are considered.

Important Note: There is a growing trend for the use of EBITDA in the eye care landscape. This is mostly driven by the influence of private equity firms looking to buyout or partner with practices. EBITDA is a non-GAAP financial calculation that is used as a valuation metric to assess the earning potential of a company. It equals the sum of net income, interest, taxes, depreciation, and amortization. This does not represent earnings or cash flow.[2] Care must be taken with its use as the methods applied for its calculation do not have a standard guideline from GAAP.

Immediate Action Items

Like the balance statement, have you recently reviewed an updated version of the practice's income statement? Obtain the latest copy available and review the document using the procedures described earlier for the balance statement. Start with large categories and gradually work your way down to the fine details. Then, ask the creator of the document for a presentation about it. Attention will, and should, first be drawn to the larger number in the statement. These are always good places to ask for more detail. Understand what comprises them as this exercise is the first step to identify and correct areas to become more profitable. For example, carefully review the COGS section. Is it accurate? Although the number may already seem high, make sure it is not missing anything. An incorrect COGS, or any other line item, may lead you to believe you are working for profit when you are losing money. Yikes!

Remember, the top line is what the practice brings in to start, and the bottom line is profit left over. Once the framework of the document is understood and you are more comfortable, critically look at what is going on throughout the company along its different arms of the business. Specifically, what are the profit margins in each area? You may be surprised to see that items that do not generate a large top line revenue end up being more profitable. This may change your priorities. With each pass through the income statement, you will notice these fine details, which will lead to even smarter questions.

Following the Cash Flow Statement

Importance

Another important financial assessment is cash flow statement. It explains the flow of cash in a business. The specifics include how exactly cash enters, where it goes, and what is left over.[1] The importance of this document is that it focuses on cash only. In business, just as in routine private life, available cash has value because it is used in exchange during transactions for goods and services.

The best way to appreciate the uniqueness of the cash flow statement is with an example. A company can have many assets of value, such as a large AR, but not have enough money available to pay its bills. It is owed a lot so it has potential money, but this is not cash on hand to be used. The results in this case is a successful business that still fails. Effective eye care providers understand the utility of each of these

Figure 9-4. Categories and organization of a cash flow statement.

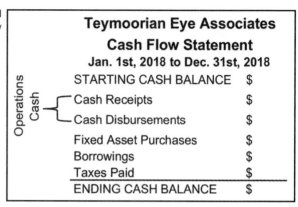

statements and their limitations when evaluating companies. It provides opportunities to improve but also protects against failure.

Keywords

Cash flow statement: A financial summary of a company that illustrates how money enters, moves, and leaves over a period of time

Positive cash flow: The state of a company where there is more cash available at the end than at the beginning, as described by the cash flow statement

Negative cash flow: The state of a company where there is less cash available at the end than at the beginning, as described by the cash flow statement

Operations cash: The amount of money generated by cash distributions subtracted from cash receipts

Cash receipts: The summation of the actual cash that is brought into a practice during the course of routine, daily operations

Cash distributions: The summation of the actual cash that leaves the practice during the course of routine, daily operations

Applications

The efficient eye care practitioner incorporates the cash flow statement to understand what is occurring to the available cash for use over a period of time. The only factors that affect the cash flow are instances when money actually comes in and leaves the company. The general formula used for it is the amount of cash available at the beginning plus the money taken in by the practice minus all the money that the practice gives away (Figure 9-4).

The activities are logged into 4 categories based upon 2 parameters. The first is if the money is coming in or out of the business. The second is whether the transaction involved occurs because of routine day-to-day activities or not. Operations cash represents the result of the daily transactions by subtracting what the practices pays out in the form of cash distributions from what it collects in cash receipts. This includes the actual payment by a patient at checkout to the practice, which exemplifies cash receipts, and the check for the phone bill that is mailed as a cash distribution.

This discussion of cash flow points out the importance of the period lengths or cycles of AR and AP. If a practice routinely gets paid by a carrier in 90 days, it shows up under AR; however, it will not physically have the cash on hand for 90 days. In the meantime, the company may need to spend money to pay bills. It has money owed to it but does not have cash readily available for utilization. This is why practices should strive to minimize their AR cycle. On the other hand, the company can extend its AP for the opposite reason. The process of lengthening AP allows cash to stay available while the company already has used the product or service from another business. The cash may have better use elsewhere for the organization until it needs to be paid out. It is important to not overextend this period of AP because it does need to be paid off at some point.

The next section of the cash flow statement includes items that are not involved in the day-to-day functions of the practice. This includes the purchase of items such as a property, building, or inventory that are needed to generate sales. These items can be categorized under fixed assets purchased. The following would be any money brought in by borrowing since it represents additional cash available to the practice. This generates positive cash flow. Another subsection is payment for income taxes for the sales generated. This creates negative cash flow. A reminder for this section, along with all of the other ones in the cash flow statement, is that money needs to be actually brought in or sent out for it to be on the statement. For example, the practice may have borrowed money, but until that cash is in hand, it will not be on the statement.

All of these components lead to the computation of the ending cash balance. It is calculated as the sum of the cash at the beginning with the operations cash along with all activities that generate positive flow and minus any with negative flow. This represents the cash readily available for use if needed. The integration of the information from this statement along with that of the balance sheet and income statement paint a clear picture of the organization's financial status. This enables the highly trained eye care provider to have a keen sense of the business aspect of the practice.[2]

Immediate Action Items

Have you seen a recent and updated cash flow statement from your practice? It is valuable to review this document to both keep you abreast of the company's actual cash and the different sources that influence it. A periodic review can shine lights on areas that need improvement by giving background knowledge about what normal figures are for each category. For example, if a reduction in cash receipts can be indictive of a change in your practice's ability to collect from AR. This may give notice that a reason exists that has disrupted its payment and is worth investigating. Like the other financial statements, take time to review your cash flow using the keywords provided previously. Repetitive assessment will allow for your continual improvement in evaluating it.

One exercise of value is appreciating the trend of your cash flow over a calendar year. Inevitably, the practice will have times of positive and negative flow. A successful practitioner and business can utilize trends in these figures to forecast for the future. This aids in operational strategy as it pertains to when money should be spent. Take a case when the practice wants to buy new equipment to upgrade what is currently used in the exam lanes. Purchasing these items at the wrong time, when the business is cash poor, may create an undesirable position of being out of money to pay for other things like payroll. If this had been delayed 1 month, it may have not been an issue at all depending on historical flow.

Valuing Money

Importance

One special topic in this section is the process of how the value of money changes over time. This is essential because the entire financial arm of an organization revolves around its worth instead of the paper it is printed on. Individuals new to business and its financial considerations have a tendency to make an incorrect assumption about monetary valuation. They assume that since the same dollar currency is used today and tomorrow that its worth is the same no matter when it is used.

The reality is what can be purchased with a dollar today is the not the same tomorrow. The buying power does not remain the same but rather fluctuates over a period of time. This variability adds complexity to the decision-making process. The elite businesses recognize this property of change and factor it into their decisions. Instead of thinking how to take action now for opportunities in the future, they put themselves in the future and determine the right steps to take in that environment. They are constantly asking if the money they are spending now is the best use of their resources.

Keywords

Inflation: An effect of decreasing the purchasing power of money or an increase in prices overall

Present value (PV): The current value of money

Future value (FV): A calculation used to determine the value of money after a certain amount of years and interest rate given a current PV

Interest: A financial operation used to describe the extra obligation incurred by borrowing a certain amount of money

Interest rate: The rate at which interest accrues

Net present value (NPV): A calculation used in evaluating investments to determine the PV based on the future value that is discounted

Internal rate of return (IRR): A method of evaluating investments by expressing how efficiently the money can be utilized

Applications

Every successful provider encounters and needs to strategically address how to improve the practice's future through investments today. This involves using its scarce resources of money. A common mistake for those that are unfamiliar with it is that the value of money today is not the same as in the future. Novices believe the math behind these evaluations are negligible, if any. They compare what the practice expects to make with the investment vs what it costs to invest.

These decisions are actually more complex. Errors in overlooking key factors can make a great investment into one that devastates the company. The silver lining is that practitioners are still capable of effectively considering these opportunities. They do so by correctly analyzing the situation through the application of fundamental concepts. This subject is the time value of money.

The discussion begins by addressing the reasons why the value of money changes over time. They are the effects of inflation, the presence of risk, and the options of opportunity costs.[1] The first is that the purchasing power of the dollar changes over time. The influence of inflation can convert the same dollar that can buy something worth $1 today to only being able to purchase something else worth .95 cents in the future. The second is the effect of risk. The different options being considered by the practitioner will typically have varying risks. It cannot be assumed that the chances of being successful are equal between placing money in high-risk, high-return stock vs a low-risk, low-reward bond. The third is that other uses for the same money exist. These situations that are not invested in are the opportunity costs.

The intelligent practitioner is able to take this complex environment and change its parameters to allow an apples-to-apples comparison between investment options. This process involves the calculation of the present value (PV) for future cash flow that would occur given the opportunity. The value created at the time of when the investment is working, known as the *future view* (FV), is discounted back to arrive at the PV. This addresses the role of interest by including the interest rate (i) and the number of years (y) involved in this process. The equation is $FV = PV \times (1 + i)^y$. All of these PVs provided by the cash flow created from the investment are added together. If the sum of the additional cash flow is greater than the amount of money needed to be invested at the beginning, the net present value (NPV) is positive and the opportunity will be fruitful. However, if the cost of investment outweighs the summation from future cash flow, the NPV is negative and the opportunity should not be undertaken.

Another method beside NPV that the practitioner may encounter is the use of internal rate of return (IRR). IRR is not the same as NPV, but both can be used during the decision-making process. The NPV gives an amount of expected value to be added while the IRR is the percentage rate of return for the investment. The IRR is calculated by setting the NPV to 0 and calculating the discount rate. Unlike the NPV that assumes one discount rate, IRR can vary and it excludes certain considerations such as the scale of the project.[2]

The smart provider uses NPV and IRR to complement one another and prevents being misled or misunderstood. For example, a small project may provide a chance for a higher return rate because of its risks or unique value. However, it may have a low NPV because of its applicability to only a small target audience.[1] In other words, there is a chance that a certain amount of people will pay a very high price for a product, but there are only a few people that would be interested in the first place.

Immediate Action Items

Do you have an upcoming project you are considering investing in for your practice? If you do not, think of one you recently did execute. Use the example to make some calculated assessments by utilizing the keywords and formulas given in this section. This will naturally lead to additional questions that you may have never carefully considered. For example, what is the current interest rate? Is that below, above, or just average? What information did the different methods reveal. Based on this and your knowledge about forecasting from your cash flow statement, it may be a good time to invest or take no action at all. This also helps to expand your thoughts on what projects your practice could possible engage in in the future and what financial implications will ensue. With practice, you will realize the more things you don't know. That is also ok. The smart person acknowledges his or her lack of wisdom. A 1000-mile journey starts with one step, which is usually the hardest of them all.

CRITICAL BUSINESS FINANCE POINTERS

* A basic, fundamental understanding of a company's key financial statements can give a clear description of how it is doing.

* Cautiously review pro forma statements as they represent estimations of the future based on the past, but they are not actual data points.

* Understand how liquid your assets are to understand just what can be turned to cash if the need arises.

* As seen on an amortization schedule, the beginning of the repayment period is when the highest percentage of a payment goes to interest as opposed to principal.

* Pay off loans with the highest interest rate first if possible.

* Do not overlook the COGS when thinking about the profitability as it can make a big difference.

* Sometimes it is more effective to reduce the COGS than increase sales. Every dollar decrease in the COGS is almost a dollar increase in sales.

* A company can have a positive net income but not have the cash needed to pay bills.

* Critical in any investment decision is to remember that the value of your dollar today is not the same as it will be tomorrow.

* Be brave and secure enough to exercise your knowledge about financial statements in your practice, but also ask professionals for clarification if something just does not seem right—it is ultimately your responsibility.

REFERENCES

1. Ittelson TR. *Financial Statements*. Pompton Plains, NJ: Career Press; 2009.
2. Harvard Business Review. *HBR Guide to Finance Basics for Managers*. Boston, MA: Harvard Business Review Press; 2012.

10

Complementing Personal Finance

Everything matters. Nothing's important.

— **Friedrich Nietzsche**

INTRODUCTION

For an eye care provider to succeed professionally in business, personal finances need to be just as equally thought-out and optimized. The study of personal finance focuses on how an individual manages his or her own financial assets. A proper understanding and application of the principles used in common personal business situations can directly be translated over into starting, growing, and maintaining an eye care practice.

Providers rely on their knowledge of personal finance in day-to-day and long-term business decisions. The following are examples of these situations: apply and paying for loans on real estate, understanding tax implications for the purchase of capital equipment, determining company sponsored retirement plans, and selecting the type of business structure for the practice. The failure to comprehend the effects of these fundamental principles in the eye care provider's personal life can cause the business to suffer. A provider cannot take care of patients and employ the staff if the front door to the office is closed. This chapter focuses on the key personal financial issues faced by a practitioner that build up to applications on the business side.

Teymoorian S. *Essential Business Fundamentals for the Successful Eye Care Practice* (pp 151-165).
© 2019 SLACK Incorporated.

What Is Personal Finance?

One area of focus that is naturally intertwined with the success of a business involves the personal financial status and acumen of its owners. The attitudes and approaches to how individuals manage their wealth remain consistent in both the business and the personal setting. Although attempts are made to keep these 2 areas of finance separate, each directly affects the well-being of the other. The best approach to deal with this complex, interdependent interaction is to begin with an understanding of fundamental finance principles. This knowledge can then be applied to common situations where decisions need to be made in both settings. The benefit to this strategy allows the individual to maximize his or her overall financial position by taking advantage of the synergy between the 2 financial arms. The whole is worth more than the sum of the parts with this practice style.

Fortunately, there are overlapping areas of wealth management from one's business and personal finance. Business owners must always have a sense of both the current and future economic environment. The decisions made today directly influence the results of tomorrow. This is exemplified by how money is actively used in the short-term setting and invested for in the long term. It is commonplace for owners to decide when and how much to allocate in these different time periods. Examples include the management of mortgages when acquiring property and the understanding of tax implications when making any financial decision.

The scope of personal finance does extend beyond these topics to include some discussion about issues that may not be emotionally easy to confront. However, these items are of critical importance and need to be addressed for the well-being of both the business and the practitioner. A responsible owner understands the uncertainty in the future and plans strategically around them to optimize their position. This process brings sensitive subjects out into the open and allows for difficult discussions to find resolutions. In the end, everyone benefits after tackling these delicate subjects.

Personal Finance in Eye Care

Successful providers take the lessons they learned to get their personal finances in order and apply a similar process to their business endeavors. The better they do personally then the more they are able invest and make solid decisions in their businesses. The valuable competencies in personal finance for the elite eye care practitioner to learn are the following: maximizing investments, optimizing mortgages, considering taxation, anticipating special circumstances, and appreciating business structures.

Maximizing Investments

Importance

One common opportunity and challenge is how to properly make investments for the future. Although an intelligent individual would be able to decipher all the information for each option and understand its repercussions, the reality is that time is limited. If the eye care provider spent all the necessary time to comprehend and evaluate these options, he would be an investor and not a doctor. This is where having trustworthy and knowledgeable individuals around can be a significant benefit. These professionals specialize in doing the due diligence that is needed and processing that information into succinct forms to be evaluated by the investor. The result is better allocation of time. The eye care practitioner is left to focus on making decisions on the larger scale.

This does not mean that the investor should be unaware and uneducated to what is occurring with his or her money by leaving all decisions to the advisors. It is the individual's responsibility for what is done at the end of the day. The eye care provider is risking hard-earned money in these investments with the hopes of making an appropriate return. An effective investor takes time to understand the basics so he or she can follow along and, more importantly, question when something seems wrong. The latter ability keeps the individual out of trouble. When in doubt, the individual does not let the pride of being a doctor disable him or her from continually learning more. This behavior avoids making poor and costly decisions.

Keywords

Personal finance: The study of an individual's management of money

Financial planner: A single or combination of advisors that help to direct an individual's financial investments in the future

Diversification: The process of spreading out investments in many forms to protect the investor in case there is a collapse in a particular market section

Asset allocation: The manner in which an investor's money is distributed between asset options

Broker: Someone that acts as a liaison in investment opportunities at the time of purchasing or selling

Securities and Exchange Commission (SEC): The US government agency in charge of protecting investors from malpractice by companies, brokers, and advisors

Mutual fund: An investment program where a combination of various stocks, bonds, and securities (portfolio) is run by a professional company on behalf of its investors

Stocks: The shares sold by a company to raise funds

Price-to-earnings (P/E) ratio: A financial calculation that relates the price of a stock to the net income earned by a firm

Performance: A description of how well an investment portfolio grew in value over a period of time

Capital gain: The profit made when an individual sells an investment

Bonds: A form of fixed-income security where a loan is made by an individual to a company with a certain term length and interest rate

Certificate of Deposit (CD): A form of fixed-income security where a loan is made by an individual to a bank with a certain term length and interest rate

Maturity: The length or point in time when payment is due

Applications

The eye practitioner's primary job is to practice medicine. Although proper education and time should be spent on personal finance matters, effective individuals understand when they need help and are humble enough to seek it out. Trustworthy financial planners add significant value by aiding the practitioner. An ideal goal is to own a group of assets that provides a good financial return but does so with minimum risk. This is achieved by diversification of the practitioner's portfolio. The individual can decide the relative risk-to-benefit strategy they want to execute. A financial planner helps with asset allocation to achieve the desired mixture. The government uses the Securities and Exchange Commission (SEC) to ensure that all these parties involved in this area are practicing within accepted guidelines.[1]

An analogy is purchasing a car. It is easy to select one when an individual has a clear understanding and desire for a particular type. This is much less obvious to those unsure of their needs and have many options from which to select. The financial planner guides the individual to what is right and creates a path to own it. The actual investing and purchasing of the assets, or car in the analogy, occurs through a broker.

The individual selects among a group of options that include stocks and bonds.[2] They can pick within these choices or obtain a combination of them through mutual funds. The latter is managed by a professional company. This helps to reduce the workload that would have been required by the individual to complete.

Stocks are a form of investment where companies exchange shares of ownership for capital. The price of the stock varies over time. There are several indices that are utilized to make decisions on which stocks to purchase. An example is the price-to-earnings (P/E) ratio that helps to understand a stock's health. The assessment for how well these investments are doing are expressed in terms of performance. The hope is to create value over a period of time that can eventually be recognized by the investor through capital gains.

Bonds and certificates of deposit (CDs) are forms of securities that are tradable financial assets. Investors use money to obtain them. At maturity, the investment is paid back along with interest. The difference between the two are typically who issues them—various institutions for bonds and banks for CDs. The date of maturity is generally longer in terms of decades for bonds and less for CDs.

Immediate Action Items

What's in your portfolio? Do you have one? If not, it is never too late to start thinking about how to get the most for the money you worked so hard to generate. Begin by considering your goals for the future such as how long you want to work, what type of lifestyle you want to lead now and in the future, and your family obligations such as your children's education. However, you should not reinvent the wheel. Ask around among your colleagues about recommendations for a great financial planner (do the same for all sorts of professionals from lawyers to plumbers). After your due diligence, select one and contact him or her for a meeting. Work together to answer questions like asset allocation and start executing on your plan. For added motivation, the sooner you start saving for things like retirement, the less negative effect it will have on your current lifestyle. For example, you will earn more interest on the dollar you invested today as opposed to one in a decade or two. Financial savvy individuals understand that they can only generate so much income from their own work. Instead, they let their money make money for them.

Optimizing Mortgages

Importance

Purchasing a home represents one of the most important investments for any individual. This venture is typically financed through a loan as most people do not have enough money saved to purchase it outright. The common misconception is that the hardest part of buying a home is locating the right one. The more difficult part is afterward with the numerous steps required to secure the needed financing via a mortgage. This challenging process, however, provides a wealth of opportunities to learn about the business world.

The successful practitioner takes advantage of this experience to benefit him- or herself, both privately and professionally. The value added to an individual's private life by owning property is obvious. Skillful management of personal investments including mortgages build equity over time by using funds that would have been spent on housing. This equity provides the investor options should he or she need to tap into it for other projects requiring funds. Another additional benefit is the improvement of the person's credit score. This helps in obtaining additional loans for private or professional reasons while minimizing the interest rates. Positive financial growth can have a snowball effect that benefits all sectors of an individual's life.

Keywords

Mortgage: The process of charging a piece of property to a creditor under the premise that the control of the property will be turned over to the debtor when payment for it is completed

Underwriting: The procedure in which a company evaluates the risk of an individual to file a claim that can either determine rates or even refuse an application

Credit report: A report of an individual's credit history that is used by lenders to evaluate a loan proposal

Consumer debt: The debt that is accumulated by an individual to acquire items that lose value or depreciate over time

Prime rate: The lowest rate of interest that can be given on loan that is generally held for those with the best credit and least risk to default

Annual percentage rate (APR): A rate representing the interest rate along with other charges

Adjustable-rate mortgage (ARM): A mortgage where the interest rate can change during the term of the loan depending on the economy

Fixed-rate mortgage: A mortgage where the interest rate remains the same through the term of the loan

Negative amortization: A situation where the repayment on a loan does not cover the cost of the interest and results in an increase in the principal balance over time

Refinancing: A financial process where an individual obtains a new mortgage with a lower interest rate to pay off his or her currently higher interest rate mortgage

Home-equity loan: A loan that can be considered as a second mortgage where the equity of an individual's home is used to obtain a loan that can be used for other immediate needs or to pay off another loan with a higher interest rate

Reverse mortgage: A financial process where a lender will pay a homeowner on a scheduled basis with cash in exchange for taking equity from the homeowner's house

Applications

The process of purchasing real estate and obtaining a mortgage is a valuable experience for the practitioner. Not only does this journey result in successful acquisition of property, but it also teaches a plethora of finance lessons. The takeaway message is to convert the knowledge gained from this experience to better situate yourself for the next opportunity.

The first step to obtaining a mortgage, after a property and creditor is selected, is underwriting. This methodical process analyzes all areas of the debtor's history with a focus on finance. This includes evaluation of current and past employment, tax filings over several years, all forms of debt including consumer debt, and credit score. The purpose of this thorough examination is to determine the risk of the individual seeking the mortgage. The creditor is in the business of making money through sound financial decisions. Lending money to a person with a high risk of defaulting is not in the lender's best interest.

If the person passes the risk test, then the interest rate is calculated. This is determined partly on credit history. The lowest rate possible, or the prime rate, is reserved for those with only excellent credit and low risk. Individuals that do not fit this ideal category have points added to the prime rate to justify the extra risk taken by the lender. These points along with other charges combine to establish the annual percentage rate (APR). The objective is to develop a strong credit history and present with the lowest risk possible to obtain a rate close to prime. The difference between mortgages of $400,000 with 3% interest rate vs 4% interest rate over 30 years is $78,000. Furthermore, mortgages can be structured as adjustable-rate or fixed-rate.

The process of paying down a mortgage involves submitting payments that cover the interest on the loan while reducing the principal. This is illustrated in an amortization schedule. At the beginning of repayment, the amount allocated to interest will be the highest. With each subsequent payment, the interest amount will decrease because the principal is reduced.[2] An ideal approach would be to pay back the loan with payments greater than the initial monthly amount, so the extra amount applies toward reducing the principal.

One special situation to avoid is negative amortization. It occurs when payments made do not cover the interest accrued. The following payment has a higher principal base leading to more interest accruing. Therefore, the remaining loan principal increases despite making payments. This is a particular concern with an adjustable-rate mortgage (ARM) as the rate is increased to a point where the resultant interest accrued surpasses the monthly payment.

There are some advantageous opportunities associated with mortgages. Certain circumstances may prevail when the borrower obtains another loan with a lower interest rate. This process of refinancing saves the borrower money over time and allows the payment amount to decrease. Another beneficial situation that may arise is if the borrower needs money on hand to pay for home repair or another investment. A home-equity loan provides that cash as the debtor borrows against the equity in the property. This is a second mortgage. An additional opportunity typically seen with elderly homeowners is a reverse mortgage. In this setting, the homeowner needs a constant stream of income because his or her retirement savings is not enough. The roles between lender and borrower are reversed. The result is that the lender pays the homeowner monthly payments but takes back ownership of the home.

Immediate Action Items

How much are you paying in interest on your mortgage? What percentage is it relative to the principal? If it is early in your repayment, sit down before you do that calculation. After the frustration of how little your money goes to reducing the principal subsides, let us think productively by assessing what can be done to place you and your family in a better financial situation. This goes back to reviewing your interest rate with what is currently available. There may be an opportunity to get a lower interest given the economic landscape. Similar to what has been discussed earlier in the book, you can pay a little more each payment period to reduce that principal faster. One strategy that helps is to convert from the traditional 24 payments per year given on the first and 15th of every month to 26 payments made every 2 weeks. Over a span of a 30-year mortgage, these 2 additional payments along with the interested saved makes a difference. It is a subtle yet meaningful change.

Another exercise is to list all of the loans you currently owe by descending order of associated interest rate. The payments to ones with the highest rates are the most inefficient uses of your money. Pay them off first with higher repayment amounts if possible. However, before you do that, use the strategies in the prior chapter about the value of money to assess if your available cash would be better off on another investment. For example, if your loan interest rates are low like 3% to 4%, you may be better off with an investment of that money that pays out 6% depending on the relative risk. The right question to ask is which one can you do more efficiently. Now think about the compounding effects of make the small changes of strategy in your life over a span of decades. Work smarter and not harder, and enjoy the extra time and money you have created.

Considering Taxation

Importance

Another critical area of finance that elite providers focus on are taxes. The broad application of tax knowledge makes it an important subject to comprehend. They play a significant role in everyone's finances including personally and professionally. It is not unusual for successful individuals to consider the tax implications for every decision they make.

The best way to deal with taxes and their effects is to understand a core set of fundamentals including their types and calculations. An easy yet financially devastating trap to fall into is being surprised by them. This occurs by not appreciating their existence given the complexity of the tax world. The consequences can be quite large and are typically uncovered later down the road. This eventual discovery compounds the issues with added penalties and fees. If these problems present at inopportune times, the effects can be disastrous. Prevention of such situations is always the easiest way to deal with them. Smart individuals have the understanding to know what they do not know and seek guidance from professionals.

Another valuable skill set to possess is comprehending how taxes are calculated. There can be meaningful advantages to knowing how personal and professional choices affect these numbers. Tax considerations can have such a huge influence that they should be acknowledged routinely in any decision-making process. Intelligent people accept that dealing with taxes is unavoidable. However, they take time to understand them to enable the selection of the best choices when situations present themselves.

Keywords

Marginal tax rate: The financial implication where the amount of tax an individual pays varies because the rate increases with additional income generated beyond certain threshold limits

Deduction: An incurred expense that can be subtracted from an individual's income to decrease the amount that is taxed

Adjusted gross income: The amount of income a person is actually taxed on, which is the total of all taxable income minus some allowable deductions

Audit: An examination from the Internal Revenue Service (IRS) to review one's financial records in order to validate an individual's tax return

Applications

Paying taxes is a necessary side effect of generating income. A common mistake many individuals commit when they initially start making a lot more money is not accounting for the amount of taxes they will owe. It is important for eye care practitioners to educate themselves on basic tax principles because it should factor into their decision-making process. Another important piece of advice is having a trustworthy accountant complete the necessary paperwork and keep the provider out of legal financial trouble. A bookkeeper also helps should there be a lot of deductions or if the provider is not efficient at maintaining records. The ideal situation is creating a productive team that brings the practitioner, accountant, and financial planner together to work in unison toward defined goals.

The first concept for the practitioner to comprehend is the tax rate. A misconception of this rate is that one number is applied to all the income produced by the individual. However, it is actually a marginal tax rate. It increases as income graduates into higher tiers. The last dollar earned in a calendar year is taxed more than the first one. As income moves up the tiers, the work required to make that additional dollar that will be kept after taxes becomes harder.

The use of deductions helps offset some of these tax implications by reducing the amount of taxable income, also known as the *adjusted gross income*. Efficient eye care providers work with their accountants to understand which items can be deducted throughout the year, and they have their bookkeeper retain a close account of them. Examples can include property taxes, charitable donations, health expenses, and transportation expenses. Another factor to consider is the type of business structure that the provider uses in the workplace. The choice made will have significant tax consequences on the individual. This will be further discussed in the next section. Again, it is important to check with a professional to understand the tax implications when making decisions that have huge financial impacts.

All of the cost and work put into accurately addressing taxes becomes invaluable should the practitioner or practice be audited. The best-case scenario is for the audit to reveal no issues. However, the provider, along with all individuals involved with the finances, will have dedicated a lot of time into the process. These are lost opportunities that could have been spent in more productive manners. The worst-case scenario in an audit could be devastating to the practitioner and the business.

Immediate Action Items

Do you think about the tax implications of every financial decision you make? With as much money on the line from a practitioner's work, it is worth your time to contemplate them. Chances are that the time you spend thinking about it will be more profitable than how much you can by working over that same period. As this thought process becomes a habit, you will appreciate more and process faster how your decisions influence the amount paid in taxes.

Where can you correctly learn what and how to think about taxes? Like you ask around for a good financial planner, perform your due diligence to locate a high-quality accountant. Not only will an accountant help with your taxes when they are due, but he or she can also be leveraged many times during the year when financial decisions need to be made. Tap into the accountant's wisdom to make smarter decisions. This practice will likely uncover more changes you can be making that you never considered. It is so important to have good people around you. Remember back to the first chapter, a great leader understands how to position individuals around him or her to maximize strengths and realizes others may be more qualified to perform certain tasks. Creating the right environment to get the most out of your supporting staff is like positioning your money to make money. Successful individuals capitalize by implementing these strategies.

Anticipating Special Circumstances

Importance

It is easy to get caught up in our busy, everyday lives at home and work. Nonetheless, it is imperative to also consider the future and plan accordingly despite these restrictions on our time available now. The reality is that no one is guaranteed tomorrow. Preparation for unexpected life changes is imperative. It is especially true for the eye care practitioner because so many other people have a dependence on him or her. Unfortunately, most wait too long and are left in a reactive mode when things occur. The result is suboptimal performance in these opportunities as they are stressful times.

Successful individuals, on the other hand, position themselves to be proactive when faced with the same challenges. They think about and prepare for such events ahead of time. Not only does this strategy decrease the emotional distress when those difficult times present, but it also provides an opportunity to maximize the outcomes. The biggest hurdle in this area arises from the uncomfortable nature of these topics. However, adult behavior is expected and proper planning should take priority. Every person owes it to him- or herself, family, and coworkers to have these difficult discussions. This demonstrates great leadership.

Keywords

Beneficiaries: The individuals that have rights to an individual's assets in the event of death

401(k): A common retirement plan provided by for-profit companies that allow employee contributions to compound over time without taxation, along with the added benefit of being exempt from federal and state taxes

Individual Retirement Account (IRA): A retirement plan that allows an individual to contribute a fixed amount of income every year that can also be tax-deductible depending on certain plans

Pension: A benefit plan given to employees by a company that provides monthly income during retirement based on how long the employee was with the company and what he or she was earning

Annuity: A financial contract where the customer can place their money to grow and compound without taxation (accumulation phase) until it is paid back to the customer with a stream of payments (annuitization phase)

Disability insurance: An insurance plan to cover lost income of an individual in the event of a disability that prevents the individual from continuing to work

Life insurance: An insurance plan that pays money to the beneficiaries of an individual in the event of death

Will: A formal document that expresses one's desire for how his or her assets will be cared for and allocated along with care for the individual's family

Estate planning: The process of thinking ahead about the structure and distribution of an individual's assets after death with a thought of attempting to minimize estate taxes

Bankruptcy: A legal procedure used by individuals and entities when they can no longer pay their debts to creditors

Applications

A practitioner has the duty to plan for life outside of and after the practice. There are a few special situations to prepare for just in case they come up. In most of these instances, the provider needs to designate beneficiaries. In any event, the time to address these contingencies is now.

The first is saving for retirement. The eye care provider, just like everyone else, hopes to have a happy retirement after having worked for many years taking care of others. Financial stability helps the transition to that stage of life. However, this does not just happen. Proper retirement planning requires thoughtful consideration and dedication. The practitioner, along with the aid of the financial planner, can work together to create goals for retirement based on the current financial situation. It is best to start as early as possible because it requires more commitment and allocation to savings later in life to accomplish the same objective. This discussion relates back to the prior section about tax implications. The successful doctor utilizes tax breaks to help invest into their retirement. This includes the use of a 401(k) and individual retirement account. A financial planner provides insightful information in this area.

The next situation is supplementing retirement funds. The hope is that the savings achieved prior to retirement will provide sufficient financial security when called upon later in life. However, additional income can be useful in retirement as well. The first is in the form of a pension. For those lucky to be in a work environment where one is offered, the extra stream of monthly cash provides support in case savings are exhausted. Another method is an annuity. This is a contract purchased from an insurance that provides regular payment back to the buyer, usually after retirement, at certain intervals. The benefit is that the value of the contract grows with interest over time, and taxes are not applied until payments are made.

Another consideration is the purchasing of insurance. The two most common types are disability and life. The purpose of these insurance plans is to provide reassurance and financial stability to the practitioner and beneficiaries when applicable. The use of disability insurance factors in if and when the provider sustains a covered injury as outlined by the plan. The restrictions on these plans vary, so it is important to be familiar with its coverage clauses. The takeaway message is that just because a person gets injured and is no longer able to work, it does not mean that the disability insurance will be valid for use.

Life insurance is the other common form of insurance related to this topic. Its purpose is to provide financial support to the provider's beneficiaries in case of death. Similar to disability insurance, not all causes of death will result in a payout. The practitioner should understand their limitations and still strive to accumulate savings that will be accessible in any circumstance despite both insurance types.

The next topic pertains to issues after death. The uncomfortableness for some individuals to discuss this matter must not prevent them for planning for it. If not done for themselves, it should be addressed for their loved ones. The writing of a will enables the practitioner to have a method to express his or her wishes after passing. Not only does this document provide insight about the person's wishes for him- or herself, but it also gives directive on how property should be allocated. This topic transitions overall to estate planning. It helps the practitioner provide additional guidance about the structure and distribution of asset allocation with strategic thought given to tax implications. This demonstrates the endless process of considering how taxes play a role in an individual's decisions, even after death.

The last subject relates to the contingency planning in case of bankruptcy. The goal is to never experience this event. However, the process of contemplating the effects of bankruptcy may provide enough awareness to help avoid it. If this situation either personally or professionally does occur, the provider must be aware of its consequences. The benefit of being knowledgeable in this subject is understanding how to turn the situation around to recovery from it. The successful eye care practitioner, including at times of failure, looks to benefit from lessons gained through experiences. Again, attitude and perception are so vital to success in both business and life.

Immediate Action Items

How will you be taking care of your beneficiaries? Have you even selected and assigned who they will be? After the obvious self-reflection needed when considering death, carefully identify your beneficiaries. This list represents the first step in effectively preparing for that time. It serves as a guide when selecting the structure and providing the detail required for dealing with life insurance, will, and estate planning. This is not a process to be rushed as it demands careful thought. However, to accomplish this goal, you need to start and work through the necessary procedures. Collaborate with your professional team already in place (ie, accountant, financial planner, and lawyer) and tackle these specifics down. You will feel much better by having the peace of mind that these decisions are behind you. It puts into perspective what is important in life and can even help to better define your business goals as well.

Appreciating Business Structures

Importance

A topic in finance that all eye care providers should be familiar with are the various business structure types that exist. The benefit of learning what options are available can help guide those that want to start a business. Successful individuals realize that to be capable to evaluate the possible options, a proper background understanding is vital. The culmination of this knowledge then allows for effective analysis and correct selection of a business structure.

The critical issue that must be addressed to appropriately complete this task is having a clear sense of organizational vision and mission. Central to these topics is properly defining its culture. Successful individuals integrate these fundamental pieces along with their business knowledge to guide their decision on company structure. The hope is to create a business that best aligns with the desired culture while achieving the goals it sets out to accomplish.

Keywords

Sole proprietorship: A business structure where the individual and his or her company are treated like a single entity with regard to taxes and liability

Limited Liability Partnership (LLP): A business structure in which more than one person runs a company but are only held to have liability to the degree in which each has invested in the group

C Corporation: A business structure where the corporation pays the taxes on earnings, but dividends are taxed at both the corporate and shareholder level

S Corporation: A business structure where the corporation is treated like a partnership, but income is passed through to shareholders and taxed only once

Applications

The simplest business structure is a sole proprietorship and serves as a good starting point. It has one owner and is not incorporated. Therefore, there is no distinction between the company and the owner. The single owner retains control over the business and its decisions. Taxes and their filings are the same as the individual's. The biggest disadvantage is that there is no personal protection with liabilities.

The least complicated option for more than one owner is a limited liability partnership (LLP). As the name states, it offers protection in the form of limited liability. Taxes are also passed through the company to the individual, only allowing taxation once. However, certain types of taxes can apply such as self-employment taxes. Shares are not issues leading to limited opportunities for growth.

The next choice is a C corporation, which represents the most common form of a corporation. It has an unlimited number of shareholders that allows for unlimited growth. When it gets large enough, it has to file with the SEC. It also provides limited liability but has tight governmental oversight. The major disadvantage is double taxation at both the corporate and individual level. However, it does permit business tax deductions.

The last option is for a C corporation to file a special subchapter S filing to convert itself to an S corporation. In an S corporation, there are less than 100 shareholders that are individuals and are all given one type of company stock. It has continued life despite a death by a shareholder and provides limited liability. A significant benefit for a S corporation are the tax considerations. It is only taxed once at the individual level as taxes are passed through the corporation without taxation. Losses can be reported on the individual's returns. The business must also closely follow rules and guidelines for tax filings to remain as an S corporation.

Immediate Action Items

Does your practice have the right business structure in place? The information and exercises throughout this book have helped you to determine where and what the company should be. Now it is time to select the appropriate structure. Work with your accountant to discuss the various options available and pick the model that aligns with our goals. You can then use the knowledge gained in this process to make better business decisions moving forward. This appreciation for the consequences from your daily choices provides a significant advantage. You will notice the complexity and identify the benefits between slightly different options. Over the span of years and decades, all of these little points add up to successfully running a business.

CRITICAL PERSONAL FINANCE POINTERS

* If you are reading this book, you should already have or be preparing your Will as you probably have dependents.
* Taking time to understand personal finance pays off twice in terms of return on investment as it naturally extends into business finance.
* Surround yourself with trustworthy professionals like a financial planner and accountant, but always put in the effort to understand at a simple level what is going on around you.
* Never be afraid to ask questions about your finances because, at the end of the day, you will have to live with the outcomes.
* Thoroughly understand the business structure you work in as it will have a significant influence on many decisions, including simple day-to-day ones.
* Think about tax implications, especially as you generate more money, because the last dollar you make in income is taxed more than the first during the year.
* Pay off debt with the highest interest first as fast as possible if the cash on hand cannot be used for another investment with a higher return.
* A method to reducing debt faster is to pay more than the scheduled payment amount in each cycle, which allows the extra amount to go directly to decreasing the remaining principal and not to interest.
* Beware of negative amortization on your mortgage where your mortgage balance can increase despite paying the required payment; this is due to higher interest rates on your ARM.
* You need to keep your consumer debt down; otherwise, you are spending money to obtain items that are losing value over time while paying it back with interest—BAD!

REFERENCES

1. Harvard Business Review. *HBR Guide to Finance Basics for Managers.* Boston, MA: Harvard Business Review Press; 2012.
2. Ittelson TR. *Financial Statements.* Pompton Plains, NJ: Career Press; 2009.

11

Utilizing Statistics

Be able to analyze statistics, which can be used to support or undercut almost any argument.

— **Marilyn vos Savant**

INTRODUCTION

There are only a few instances when anyone has all the information needed to make a decision. The choices made by an eye care practitioner are no different. However, the lack of data does not mean that informed decisions cannot be reached during the process. The proper use of statistics can provide the necessary support in these uncertain times. Statistics is the collection and use of data to aid in the selection of the best option. The successful provider understands how and when to incorporate this science to excel in business.

The application of statistics can be used in all aspects of business. The practitioner encounters it numerous times throughout the day. Obvious examples include areas where numbers are frequently used such as in finance with return on investments and negotiations with reservation points. The extent of statistics does not end there. In fact, statistical theories and methods are also evident in human resources with employee reviews and marketing with website analytics. It is in these unexpected areas that the incorporation of statistics creates a strategic advantage to the user over the competition.

This chapter takes a logical approach to the use of statistics in the life of eye care practitioners. The first section lays the basic groundwork to be used throughout the rest of the discussion. This leads to sections where various real-life situations are presented along with different types of statistics that can be applied to make the best

Teymoorian S. *Essential Business Fundamentals for the Successful Eye Care Practice* (pp 167-177).
© 2019 SLACK Incorporated.

decisions. The aim is to orient doctors with sound statistical theories to employ in day-to-day activities where these decisions can significantly impact the practice.

What Is Statistics?

Solid decision making in any venture requires the ability to effectively take information that is gathered and use it in a strategic manner to make choices. This premise assumes that the underlying facts are accurate and correctly represent the desired data to be analyzed. The entire process falls apart without reliable information. Simply stated, garbage in equals garbage out.

However, it should not be assumed that all information can be lumped into either being good or bad. The reality is that most information is useful if its parameters are understood and applied properly into a given situation.[1] The best analogy is that sometimes a cut just needs a bandage, but in other instances, it is best to use sutures. The ability to gather and understand data for applications in decision-making situations can make the difference between success and failure.

The pressing issue becomes why we even need to go through this exercise to obtain data to run statistics in the first place. All the necessary information can be obtained and an intelligent decision can be made if enough time and effort is used. Although in theory it makes sense to wait until a complete set of data is available, the reality is that this either is not possible to do or would be so laborious to deem it cost ineffective. The value of statistics becomes evident when given these constraints on data collection. Statistics allows the use of collected information from an appropriate sample from a larger group to make educated decisions about the entire targeted population.

The takeaway is that statistics, if understood and used properly, can support or detract from a choice when confronted with options in a given situation. Furthermore, a clear understanding of the different statistical calculations and their applications help the decision makers remain flexible to the various situations that might be presented. This thoughtful analysis allows the best use of their resources (bandage or sutures) to address their needs.

Statistics in Eye Care

The value of statistics in eye care is illustrated by the fundamental role that numbers play in the decision-making process for any organization. Accurately collecting data and thoughtfully generating key numbers differentiates a company from its competitors. The former is a time-tested organization that continually improves by making solid choices based on facts. The latter is an underachieving company that learns from making costly mistakes first by relying on emotions. Successful eye care practitioners need to demonstrate the following capabilities in statistics: understanding basic statistics, using parametric testing, identifying non-parametric testing, and applying regression analysis.

Understanding Basic Statistics

Importance

Understanding numbers and their applications through statistical analysis is a required skill set for any successful person. In particular, the use of statistics allows individuals to rely on what is truly happening in a situation instead of being influenced by emotions. The capability to separate factual information from those affected by feelings allows practitioners and their businesses to make less mistakes. It avoids knee-jerk reactions in challenging situations while fostering a more logical and calmer approach to problem solving.

The best companies utilize these objective metrics to be more efficient and effective throughout their organizations. A strong knowledge in this discipline also enables a thoughtful critique of how numbers are derived. This prevents the problems from trusting misleading information and identifies areas of limitations that need to be considered when assessing situations.

Keywords

Statistics: The study of the collection and analysis of data

Descriptive statistics: A type of statistics that describes the collected data set used for analysis

Discrete: A data point that has a limited number of possible values

Continuous: A data point that has an infinite number of possible values

Graphical method: The use of graphs to represent data

Numerical method: The use of numbers to represent data

Mean: A method to calculate an average of a data set by adding the values of the data points and dividing by the number of data points

Median: A method to calculate an average of a data set by sequencing the data points in numerical order and then picking the number in the middle of the group

Mode: A method to calculate an average of a data set by selecting the value that appears the most

Range: A description of a data set that is defined by its extreme values

Standard deviation: A description of a data set that expresses the degree to which there is dispersion of the set's values

Variance: A description of a data set that is the mean of the squared distances for each point to the population's mean

Distribution: The way in which the data points are spread out

Normal distribution: A traditional or bell spread of a distribution

Skew distribution: A loop-sidedness of a distribution

Percentile: A measure in statistics in which a given percentage of data points fall below or above a certain value

Probability: A measurement in statistics to describe the odds of an event occurring

Combinations: The number of ways objects from a set can be grouped together regardless of the order

Permutations: The number of ways objects from a set can be grouped together where the order does matter

Applications

Statistics are utilized in a wide range of medical and business applications. The type of statistics selected in a given situation will be affected by what information is available. The validity and subsequent usefulness of the resulting calculations depends on the accuracy of the data points measured and collected. The successful eye care practitioner understands these fundamental properties of statistics and strategically applies them in the right conditions.

The effective use of statistics begins with a characterization of the data set that is obtained. This is known as *descriptive statistics*. The data points can be discrete or continuous, and expressed in a graphical and numerical methods. Examples of these would be to either plot out the intraocular pressure (IOP) readings from one patient on a graph or write them out, respectively.

A useful calculation to describe the data set is the average for the group of values. This meaning of average, however, can take on several meanings. It is important to understanding what type of calculation was used to determine that number. This is especially true if this information will be used to make a decision because it can change the choice that is selected. Consider the following list of IOP readings in mm of mercury placed in ascending order from a patient after he is started on a prostaglandin analogue: 12, 12, 12, 13, 15, 15, 16, 16, and 17. The mean is 14, median is 15, and mode is 12. Each of these can be stated as the average but can characterize the data set in a different manner. The consequence is that there can be a misinterpretation of what is meant by average. This can lead to a suboptimal decision.

Additional statistics about this data set could provide the practitioner more information that can be valuable in certain settings. This includes the range, which is 12 to 17, the standard deviation is 1.9, and the variance is 3.9. These calculations provide sophistication to the average. The range provides the minimum and maximum values with which the IOP has been measured. The standard deviation gives an idea of how deviated each measurement is from the mean, or in other ways, how close they are to the mean. The variance provides an understanding of how much variability is in the measurements.

A smaller standard deviation translates to most measurements being near the mean, and a smaller variance expresses less variability between numbers. In this situation, it means the IOPs are close to the mean and do not vary much. A larger standard deviation and variance represents a large spread of numbers away from the mean and different from one another. This is useful information for the provider to know beyond just the mean IOP.

Another approach to interpret this information is to view its distribution. In a normal distribution, the values follow a traditional bell curve with most numbers near the center and tapering off in both directions. Sometimes these numbers do

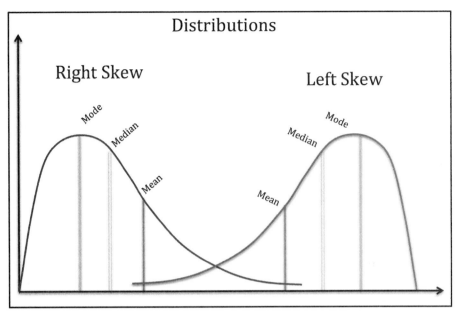

Figure 11-1. Visual representation of the different types of averages.

not follow such a balanced distribution and can appeared to have a skew distribution (Figure 11-1). This influences the mean, median, and mode. A different view of this information is to examine the numbers by percentile. This application provides the practitioner an idea of which IOP values are grouped together when the numbers are broken up into percentage groups. For example, the top 25% had IOPs of 16 to 17. The bottom 50% had values of 12 to 15.

A few other descriptive statistics are useful to the eye care provider. The first is probability, which is the likelihood of an event occurring. The most common application is the *P* value in research. A *P* value of less than 0.05 represents the chances that the observed findings in an experiment occurring due to chance is less than 5%. This is typically deemed statistically significant.

The next concepts are combinations and permutations. These relate to how many ways things can be combined, with the order not being relevant in combinations while being important in permutations. An example in an eye care practice is to consider a situation where there is a group of 6 receptionists, 13 technicians, and 4 doctors. The number of combinations is simply how many different ways a group, with one type of employee, can sit in 3 chairs. The number of permutations is how many groups are possible but with one of each type sitting in a particular order of chairs. There are 312 combinations and 1,872 permutations. These and the following medical applications of statistics can be transferred over to business-related uses. The takeaway is to understand the underlying principles and their limitations.

Immediate Action Items

How comfortable are you with using statistics in your practice? For some people, just the thought of numbers and math make them sweat. If you feel that way, then take time to review again and practice exercises to master the basic topics discussed in this section. Remember, you do not need advanced knowledge in this area as you can always have professional help if that time comes. However, you should be able to utilize simple knowledge to assess the validity and analyze the numbers around you. The time spent on jumping past this mental hurdle will be well worth it, both as a doctor and businessperson.

Using Parametric Testing

Importance

The most intuitive thoughts on how to use statistics involves taking measurements and processing them to generate thoughtful analysis. This approach provides factual information about a situation that can guide businesses to determine their course of action. The importance of possessing this ability is that usually all the information about a targeted group cannot be obtained. The successful individual harnesses statistics to understand the whole from an analysis of one part of it. This in turn aids in the decision-making process.

The ability to perform this task successfully includes 2 critical steps. The first is that the data collected need to be accurate and meaningful. This valued information provides the solid support on which to build. A common mistake is the thought that this infrastructure will not be tested over time. This belief arises from complacency that individuals can have by thinking that numbers are 100% accurate and will not be questioned. In reality, successful individuals routinely will ask for specifics on data collection to validate the numbers and avoid a possible source of error or be misled. This behavior allows them to not only continually learn but also critically assess the provided information.

The second step is selecting the right analysis to perform on the gathered information. The large diversity of options can initially overwhelm those unfamiliar with them. This leads certain individuals to step back and passively accept the interpretation provided to them. Although having a masterful understanding on statistics would be perfect, in actuality, the requirement to be successful is less stringent. The key features are the appreciation that this variety exists and ability to correctly select the best analysis for a given situation. The rest is the application of the data to generate results. This process then either supports or opposes a proposed solution for a given situation.

Keywords

Parametric statistics: Statistics that have a fixed number of parameters that assume the sample from the population follows a probably distribution

Population: A set that has all the data points of a group

Sample: A set that has a fraction of all the data points of a group

Central limit theorem: A theory in statistics where the mean of a large group of variables will have a normal distribution even if the distribution of its smaller groups is not

Hypothesis: A proposed explanation of observations based on limited information

Null hypothesis (H_0): A hypothesis that the observations noted have occurred by chance events

Alternative hypothesis (H_1): A hypothesis that the observations noted did not occur by chance events

T-test: A statistical test that assesses if 2 sets of data are significantly different from each other

T-score: Standardized scores used in statistics

P value: A calculated value of probability typically used in hypothesis testing to quantify the likelihood of an event or its extreme occurring when the null hypothesis is correct

Analysis of variance (ANOVA): A calculation to describe the degree in which 2 or more groups vary from one another

Applications

Parametric statistics allow the practitioner to evaluate situations where the parameters of a situation are set and the assumptions are customary. An application of this is seen with hypothesis testing. The structure beings by stating the null hypothesis (H_0), which expresses that no difference exists between the mean of the sample from that of the population. The alternative hypothesis (H_1) states that there is a difference. Then, a P value is selected to appropriately describe the level of certainty that is desired. The analysis can then be performed using a t-test to determine a t-score. This information will either support or oppose the null hypothesis. A similar approach can then be taken to evaluate the variation between 2 or more groups by using analysis of variance (ANOVA).

Examples of these uses are abundant in clinical research that the eye care practitioner is exposed to routinely. The successful practitioner takes those principles and applies them in business situations to understand them and make decisions. This includes assessing whether the pay salary for the technician core at one practice is different from the population, or if there is a difference between 2 independent practices.

Immediate Action Items

Do you have a question in mind facing your practice where statistical analysis may help in the decision making? Chances are that they exist. Select one and attempt to run through it as an exercise based on the keywords discussed. Although you may need additional information or a statistical textbook, the goal is to start thinking in a more pragmatic manner. This will help you convert your real-life problem to one that can be assessed and supported through statistics.

Identifying Non-Parametric Testing

Importance

There are instances when an assessment needs to be performed, but there cannot be an assumption that the population follows a probably distribution. Also, the number of parameters may be increasing or decreasing. This situation does not excuse the necessity to still make effective decisions. Intelligent individuals expand their statistic capabilities to fill this void or seek professional advice when needed. The same criteria for obtaining useful parametric statistics also applies in these non-parametric cases. The importance of proper care of data collection and appropriate analysis usage cannot be understated. This enables businesses that are willing to embrace statistics to possess a competitive advantage that differentiates them from the competition.

Keywords

Non-parametric statistics: Statistics where assumptions to the population distribution cannot be made and the number of parameters can change

Mann-Whitney U test: A non-parametric statistic used to determine if 2 sample means from a population are equal or not

Wilcoxon Signed Rank test: A non-parametric statistic used to test if 2 dependent samples were taken from a population of the same distribution

Applications

Situations that do not have a set number of parameters or routine distributions require a different type of statistical analysis. The challenge is how to generate useful information in this setting. There are several methods that can be applied depending on the circumstances and what is hoped to be accomplished from the analysis. Two in particular are the Mann-Whitney U test and Wilcoxon Signed Rank test. Following is a discussion of each, along with a medical example. Their principles can then be transferred over to applications in the business setting.

The first is a Mann-Whitney U test. This is similar to the Wilcoxon Rank Sum test that can take the place of an unpaired t-test. However, it should not be mistaken for the Wilcoxon Signed Rank Sum test, which involves paired testing. The Mann-Whitney U test attempts to determine if 2 samples came from the same population. In hypothesis testing, it would support the null hypothesis that they are the same or, alternatively, that they are different. The assumptions it makes is that the distribution of the 2 samples are similar. An example would be to evaluate if there is age difference of when patients with primary open angle glaucoma and pseudoexfoliation glaucoma are diagnosed. A data set is collected, including the age at diagnosis for a group of each type. The data are computed and analyzed for statistical significance to determine if an age difference exists with these 2 groups.

The next one is a Wilcoxon Signed Rank test. The goal is to determine if 2 samples were taken from a population with similar distributions. It does not assume a normal population. It requires pairs of ranked data sets that are random and ordinal. An example would be determining if there is a difference in the length of drug effectiveness for decreasing IOP between 2 medications. The data set of how long the drops were able to maintain lower pressures are compared and ranked. The resulting computation would like support or oppose a difference among the drops.

Immediate Action Items

Are you dealing with an issue that requires skills beyond basic statistics? The key is to understand that your problem would benefit from the aid of professionals. Like other areas in practice, it is ok to seek the help of others with experience. You probably would not try to complete your own complex tax returns, so ask a statistician for guidance when needed. Not only can they lead you to an answer, but they also ask thought-provoking questions along the way you may have never considered. This will enhance your ability to evaluate other situations in the future. Gaining knowledge is a gradual process, so strive to get better every day, even it is just a little bit at a time.

Applying Regression Analysis

Importance

Regression analysis is a statistical calculation that demands special attention given its frequent use. Successful eye care practitioners routinely encounter situations where its utilization is applicable in the private and professional setting. The ability to understand the dependence between 2 variables has many uses. Some areas in practice that benefit from its knowledgeable use include operations, human resources, and economics. Following the theme discussed throughout this chapter, the businesses that excel are those that are able to appropriately use statistics to make well-informed decisions.

Keywords

Regression analysis: A model in statistics to estimate the relationships of 2 variables

Regression: The relationship of one dependent variable relative to changes with independent variables

Dependent variable: A variable where its value does rely on the value of another variable

Independent variable: A variable where its value does not rely on the value of another variable

Correlation: The relationship between variables

Correlation coefficient: The linear dependence of 2 variables through the use of a number between -1 and +1

Applications

Regression analysis serves as a modeling theory used in forecasting that can be especially valuable in process-oriented positions such as operations. This form of analysis studies the regression between a dependent and independent variable.

In other words, it determines how much of a change in the dependent variable would occur with a particular change in the independent variable. This assumes that the other independent variables are held constant. The result is a process to assess the correlation between variables, which can be expressed through a correlation coefficient.

An example would be to study the relationship between the number of patients seen and the amount of revenue generated in the office. The independent variable is the number of patients (x axis) and the dependent variable is the revenue (y axis). Data points are plotted on the graph and a best-fit line is determined. The result is measurement of correlation. This information can then be applied to optimizing patient load and scheduling ancillary staff according to the number of doctors used to see the patients.

Immediate Action Items

Are you considering whether to add another doctor or even expand your office to generate more profit? A core part of this decision should be based on statistics to provide the data you need to move forward. A regression analysis can help. Consider all of the variables involved, both dependent and independent. Using the keywords provided along with a statistical textbook or guide, practice running a regression analysis on the issue. As you practice and think about the problem more, you will begin to recognize what variables matter most and how they affect the desired results. This will shine light back to your operations and how processes are being managed. You may arrive at a solution where, given the amount of office space and providers, the practice needs more technicians above anything else. Utilize statistics to model these situations and allow that information to support your decisions.

CRITICAL STATISTICS POINTERS

* Useful data are required to calculate useful statistics; garbage in equals garbage out.
* A clear understanding and use of statistics can help make decisions that give us the best chance to succeed.
* If a particular type of statistic is used, make sure to know its limitations to be aware for when it may fail.
* Identifying and acquiring the right sample leads to better forecasts when relying on these data.

* A solid foundation in statistics enhances many operational applications.
* A successful individual that has a subtle understanding of statistics sniffs out mistakes that can turn out to be very costly if not addressed.
* The use of statistics should support but not solely make a business decision because it does not take into account some intangible aspects of business.

REFERENCE

1. Berman K, Knight J, Case J. *Financial Intelligence, Revised Edition: A Manager's Guide to Knowing What the Numbers Really Mean*. Boston, MA: Harvard Business Review Press; 2013.

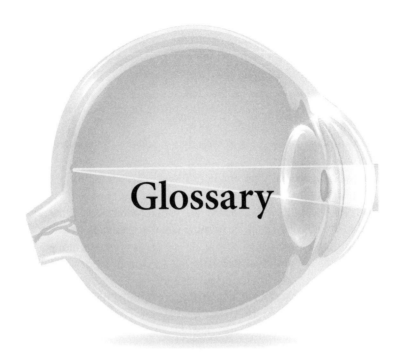

Glossary

A

Ability: An employee's aptitude for performing a single or set of tasks

Absenteeism: The repetitive nature of unexcused absence from work

Accounts payable (AP): A collection of bills or credits a company owes another party that needs to be paid

Accounts receivable (AR): A collection of payments that are owed to the company

Accrued expenses: The money a company owes for expenses it has accumulated over time

Accumulated depreciation: The total depreciation collected since the acquisition of an asset

Achievements: A list of accomplished goals that are typically difficult to reach and warrant recognition

Acquisition: The business process where one company takes over another one

Actions: The coordination of tasks to execute a strategy

Add-on: The addition of extra software or devices to a company's core IT equipment to increase or improve its current system

Adjustable-rate mortgage (ARM): A mortgage where the interest rate can change during the term of the loan depending on the economy

Teymoorian S. *Essential Business Fundamentals for the Successful Eye Care Practice* (pp 179-202).

Adjusted gross income: The amount of income a person is actually taxed on, which is the total of all taxable income minus some allowable deductions

Affective commitment: An employee's decision to remain with a company based on emotional connection

Affirmative action: A policy that favors the hiring of individuals from previously discriminated groups

Alternative hypothesis (H_1): A hypothesis that the observations noted did not occur by chance events

Alternative to a negotiated agreement (ATNA): The alternative a party has if a negotiated agreement does not occur

Americans With Disabilities Act (ADA): A law that protects the rights of those with physical and mental disabilities to be granted equal access to jobs and services

Amortization schedule: A schedule that shows the breakdown of a payment for a loan over its payback period that illustrates the amount of money that goes interest and principal

Analysis of variance (ANOVA): A calculation to describe the degree in which 2 or more groups vary from one another

Anchoring: The process of achieving a desired result by strategically beginning at a more advantageous starting point

Annual percentage rate (APR): A rate representing the interest rate along with other charges

Annuity: A financial contract where the customer can place their money to grow and compound without taxation (accumulation phase) until it is paid back to the customer with a stream of payments (annuitization phase)

Asset: A valued resource owned by a company

Asset allocation: The manner in which an investor's money is distributed between asset options

Assumptions: The beliefs one holds about the other side and its issues

Atmosphere: The feeling and image that is created in an office based on design and decorations

Attributes: The qualities or traits of a person

Audit: An examination from the Internal Revenue Service (IRS) to review one's financial records in order to validate an individual's tax return

Awareness gap: The space between what consumers know about a company's products and services vs what is really offered

B

Background check: A review of a potential employee's history for disciplinary action

Backward pass analysis: A critical path diagram evaluation that estimates time on the basis of when steps can occur at the latest moment without interfering with the timing of a process

Bad debt: A debt that is owed but cannot be recovered

Balance sheet: A financial statement for a company that provides a detailed breakdown of how it is composed at one particular instant in time using assets, liabilities, and shareholders' equity

Bankruptcy: A legal procedure used by individuals and entities when they can no longer pay their debts to creditors

Banner ads: An advertisement placed on websites that are routinely seen at the top of the page

Banners: An advertisement placed at the physical location of a company

Behavioral style: A slow thought process that bases decisions on how it will influence others

Benchmarking: An analysis where the performance of a process is compared to a standard

Beneficiaries: The individuals that have rights to an individual's assets in the event of death

Best alternative to a negotiated agreement (BATNA): The best ATNA a party has in a negotiation

Blog: An online form of writing about a topic in an informal manner

Body language: The unspoken expressions of emotions and thoughts based on body positioning and behavior

Bonds: A form of fixed-income security where a loan is made by an individual to a company with a certain term length and interest rate

Book value: The value of something as documented in the financial books of a company

Bottleneck: The rate-limiting step in a process

Bottom line: The amount of revenue left over after all costs and expenses are accounted (synonymous with *profit, income,* and *earnings*)

Bounce rate: A percentage used to describe the effectiveness of a website to keep the attention of the viewer, which is measured by the number of viewers that enter and leave the site quickly as opposed to those that stay and browse

Brainstorm: The process of discussing issues and allowing the individuals of the group to generate possible solutions

Brand equity: The value of a brand based on consumer perception as opposed to the actual goods and services

Brand identity: The unique characteristics of a product or service as created by the company

Brand recall: A measure of how well consumers relate a brand to its class of products

Break-even (BE) point: The evaluation to determine the sales volume needed to have the total costs equal the total revenue

Brick and mortar: A physical building for a company

Broker: Someone that acts as a liaison in investment opportunities at the time of purchasing or selling

Bullwhip effect: A phenomenon that demonstrates inefficiencies in supply chain management based on forecasts of demand where the effects are most noted later in a process

Burnout: An extreme condition in which employees have exhausted their ability to properly work anymore

Business finance: The study of a company's management of money

Business model: A concept that is structured with guidelines on how to run the operations of a business

Business plan: The way in which a business model is executed

Business–value-added (BVA): An expenditure of a resource during a process that does not increase the value of the product or service but does provide benefit to the business and its processes

Buttons: A graphical interface on a website that creates an action when clicked

C

C Corporation: A business structure where the corporation pays the taxes on earnings, but dividends are taxed at both the corporate and shareholder level

Calls to action: A method to increase leads on a website where interactivity between the viewer and website results in additional actions that is of interest to the viewer

Capacity: The highest output that can be achieved in a particular process over a certain time without any constraints on the pathway

Capital gain: The profit made when an individual sells an investment

Capital stock: The stock held by owners that represents the money needed to begin and add onto a business

Cash: The most liquid form of money

Cash distributions: The summation of the actual cash that leaves the practice during the course of routine, daily operations

Cash flow statement: A financial summary of a company that illustrates how money enters, moves, and leaves over a period of time

Cash receipts: The summation of the actual cash that is brought into a practice during the course of routine, daily operations

Cause-related event marketing: Company advertisement done at an event that promotes a cause

Centers for Medicare & Medicaid Services (CMS): The US federal agency that manages Medicare and also coordinates at the state level to provide Medicaid

Central limit theorem: A theory in statistics where the mean of a large group of variables will have a normal distribution even if the distribution of its smaller groups is not

Certificate of Deposit (CD): A form of fixed-income security where a loan is made by an individual to a bank with a certain term length and interest rate

Champion: An employee or customer that strongly believes in and promotes a company

Character: The summation of a person's values, beliefs, and attributes

Chief Executive Officer (CEO): The C-Suite individual and highest-ranked employee that has the final say over all matters within a company

Chief Financial Officer (CFO): The C-Suite individual that oversees all financial issues

Chief Informational Officer (CIO): The C-Suite individual that manages the information technology

Chief Medical Officer (CMO): The C-Suite individual responsible for medical matters

Chief Operating Officer (COO): The C-Suite individual that governs operations

Chief-Suite (C-Suite): The aggregate of executive-level individuals within an organization

Churn rate: The percentage of customers that stop buying a product or using a service from a company

Climate: A set of internal, short-term perceptions of individuals about an organization based on the current management and leadership styles, or external ones dependent on the effects from outside competition

Closed-ended question: A style of question where answered require simple responses like "Yes" or "No"

Combinations: The number of ways objects from a set can be grouped together regardless of the order

Common stock: A rudimentary type of stock that offers its owners the lowest rights, including the receipt of dividends when offered or assets should the company be liquidated

Communication skills: The ability to listen and respond to others

Community event marketing: Company advertisement done at an event held for the community, which is usually near the physical location of business

Compensation: The manner in which an employee is paid for his or her work

Competencies: The summation of an employee's abilities and skill set

Competitive landscape: An analysis that first identifies and understands the competitors in a desired marketplace, and then performs a self-evaluation for strengths and weaknesses to guide positioning for success in that space

Complements: A relationship between 2 products where an increase in the price of one leads to increase in the demand for the other

Compliance: The set of decisions made and actions performed to follow required rules and regulations

Comprehensive Performance Review (CPR): A formal evaluation process where an employee's performance is evaluated and goals are set for the future

Comptroller: The individual responsible for a company's accounting (synonymous with *controller*)

Computer-based training: The use of computers as a medium to provide educational material to users

Conceptual style: A thought process that bases decisions on its effect on larger-scale themes

Confidentiality: The condition of keeping secret or private (synonymous with *privacy*)

Conflict of interest: The condition that exists when the actions of one individual might be affected by outside influences that provide benefit to the individual for a particular behavior

Conflict resolution: The process of identifying and addressing problems between individuals

Consumer debt: The debt that is accumulated by an individual to acquire items that lose value or depreciate over time

Content: The information presented on a company's website

Continuance commitment: An employee's decision to remain with a company based on the degree of difficulties that would arise from changing employment

Continuous: A data point that has an infinite number of possible values

Controller: The individual responsible for a company's accounting (synonymous with *comptroller*)

Conversion rate: The percentage of viewers entering a website that will produce a desired result, such as purchasing a product or service

Copyright: The legal right of an owner over literature, artwork, or music

Corrective action: A guideline given by a supervisor to an employee as a means to make changes based on evaluations of the employee's performance

Correlation: The relationship between variables

Correlation coefficient: The linear dependence of 2 variables through the use of a number between -1 and +1

Cost: The amount of money needed to create a product that was sold

Cost of fixed assets: The collection of property and equipment owned and used by the practice for its routine operations

Cost of goods sold (COGS): The cumulative costs incurred by a company to directly create the products that are sold

Counseling: A process where a supervisor and employee discuss the employee's behavior and actions with a focus on guidance for the employee on areas of improvement to better achieve goals

Creative process: A marketing approach to foster the development and execution of a thought or strategy for a product or service

Credit limit: The maximum amount of credit a company can utilize from a given financial agreement, like a line of credit

Credit report: A report of an individual's credit history that is used by lenders to evaluate a loan proposal

Critical path diagram: An algorithm that depicts how the order of steps in a process can be arranged with the goal of best optimizing time

Cross-functional training: A style of training where individuals gain the necessary skills and abilities to perform, not only their own duties, but also those of other team members in different roles

Cross-promotion: The use of one product or service in a company's portfolio to introduce and promote another to a customer

Culture: The long-term image and behavior of an organization that is exemplified by leadership and seen as the appropriate way for employees to conduct themselves

Current assets: A collection of assets that will routinely be converted to cash within the next year, including cash on hand, accounts receivable, inventory, and prepaid expenses

Current debt: The amount owed in loans that need to be repaid in less than 1 year

Customer perception: The feelings and thoughts consumers have for a company's brand and its category

Customer profile: The characteristics of a company's targeted customer

Customer ratings: The grading of a company's products and services

Cycle time: The length of time from the end of having one thing being completed in a process to the next thing being finished

D

Dashed line: A type of line used in organizational charts denoting functional authority to give tasks to others, but not as a direct supervisor

Data archiving: The migration of data from one computer to either another computer or storage medium

Data integration: The process where information from various sources are brought together

Data migration: The process where information is moved from one source to another

Data sanitization: The process of converting data containing sensitive material to a safer form that can be distributed

Debt: The condition of owing something to another person, business, or institute

Debt-to-equity ratio: A representation of how much money a company owes in debt relative to the amount of investor equity

Deduction: An incurred expense that can be subtracted from an individual's income to decrease the amount that is taxed

Define-Measure-Analyze-Improve-Control (DMAIC) process: A series of steps used to evaluate and improve a process

Demographics: The statistical information of a group, which is usually that of the target audience

Dependent variable: A variable where its value does rely on the value of another variable

Depreciation: A term used to express the decrease in value of an asset over time due to natural wear and tear from use

Descriptive statistics: A type of statistics that describes the collected data set used for analysis

Development: A process of improvement through learning, experiencing, and maturing

Direct report: A type of reporting in an organization where one individual is immediately in charge of another one

Directive style: A fast thought process that bases decisions on information in order to proceed to the next topic

Director: An employee with an elevated position and responsibility for the overall direction of a given arm within a business (and not the actual execution of the plan, which is left to the supervisors and managers)

Disability insurance: An insurance plan to cover lost income of an individual in the event of a disability that prevents the individual from continuing to work

Discrete: A data point that has a limited number of possible values

Discrimination: The unfair treatment of one or a group of individuals based on age, sex, or race

Diseconomies of scale: The condition where long-term costs increase as output increases

Distribution: The way in which the data points are spread out

Diversification: The process of spreading out investments in many forms to protect the investor in case there is a collapse in a particular market section

Diversity: A quality of having a mixture of backgrounds, values, and beliefs that can help provide advantages that could not be achieved with a more homogenous set of individuals

Dividends: An amount of money paid by a company to its shareholders based upon profitability

Domain name: A company's website address

Dotted line: A type of line used in organizational charts denoting authority to only give advice to an individual

Downtime: A time when either a step or the entire process cannot occur for a particular reason

Downward communication: An organizational communication style where information is transferred from the top of a hierarchy to the bottom

E

Earnings: The amount of revenue left over after all costs and expenses are accounted (synonymous with *profit*, *income*, and *bottom line*)

Earnings before interest, taxes, depreciation, and amortization (EBITDA): A non-GAAP calculation used to assess the financial performance of a business to assess its earning potential

Economics: The study of how scarce resources are utilized in society

Economies of scale: The condition where long-term costs decrease as output increases

Elasticity: The degree of responsiveness

Electronic data interchange (EDI): The exchange of data between 2 computers or networks

Electronic faxing (e-faxing): The act of using a computer system to transmit faxes

Electronic health record (EHR): A medical record that is in electronic form (synonymous with electronic medical record or EMR)

Electronic medical record (EMR): A medical record that is in electronic form (synonymous with electronic health record or EHR)

Electronic prescriptions (e-prescriptions or eRx): The act of using a computer system to prescribe medications for a patient from a doctor to a pharmacy

Electronic referrals (e-referrals): The act of using a computer system to create, submit, and obtain referrals from one party to another

Employee investment: The belief that when employees are given the opportunity to take part in the steps of addressing a problem that they will be motivated to see its success

Empowerment: The act of giving support and providing autonomy to an individual or group that allows them to make and follow through on their own decisions

Encryption: The process of safe-guarding sensitive data by converting them into code with the goal to prevent unauthorized access

Entry-level position: A low-level role in an organization where an employee without much experience first begins in a particular field of work

Equilibrium: The price at which supply equals demand

Equity theory: A method of employee thinking that uses the treatment of others as a reference point on how appropriately the individual is being treated in an organization

Estate planning: The process of thinking ahead about the structure and distribution of an individual's assets after death with a thought of attempting to minimize estate taxes

Evaluation: A process where the job performance of an employee is reviewed and rated

Executive position: A high-level role in an organization where an employee with management experience can plan and direct actions on a grand scheme

Expanding the pie: The procedure to identify and enlarge the benefits of all issues in a negotiation to create more value for each side based on their priorities

Expense: The amount of money spent to provide the ancillary support needed to create a product that was sold such as marketing, research, and administrative

Expertise: The quality of having experience in an area or field

Export: A good produced inside of a nation but sold outside of it

External environment: The happenings and atmosphere outside an organization

External marketing: Marketing to those outside of an organization

F

Feedback: A part of the evaluation process where an employee's areas of strengths and weaknesses are discussed, along with recommendations for improvement

Financial Accounting Standards Board (FASB): An organized group of business professionals, including accountants, that provides the standards for financial accounting through the use of GAAP

Financial planner: A single or combination of advisors that help to direct an individual's financial investments in the future

First-to-market: The condition of being the first product or service to be offered for a certain category

Fishbone diagram: A cause-and-effect schematic representation that lists all possible sources of error that can help identify the problem with the hopes of localizing the causative issue

Fixed cost: A cost that does not vary regardless of the output quantity created

Fixed-rate mortgage: A mortgage where the interest rate remains the same through the term of the loan

Flagging: The act of highlighting data or a process to make it easily identifiable when needed such as in a review process

Flexibility: The ability to change and be dynamic based upon current conditions

Flow time: The length of time needed for one thing to go from the beginning to the end of a process

Forecasting: An exercise in predicting the future based on historical data

Formal training: The official process where an employee in a new role is trained on how to properly perform the expected duties

Formalization: The degree in which an organization is run by official rules of conduct and behavior

Forward pass analysis: A critical path diagram evaluation that estimates time on the basis of when steps can occur at the earliest times to complete a process

Framing: The action of positioning a thought or action in a particular way to associate it with a desired effect

Full-time equivalent (FTE): A method to denote the expected work from a hire where this information aids in the measuring of employee production and for allocation of budgets

Future value (FV): A calculation used to determine the value of money after a certain amount of years and interest rate given a current PV

G

Game theory: The study of human behavior when placed in strategic situations like games

Gantt chart: A schematic used to illustrate when each part of a process will start and end relative to each other

Generally accepted accounting principles (GAAP): A collection of accepted accounting rules and guidelines set forth by the Financial Accounting Standards Board

Go-live: A specific point in time during the implementation process when actions performed on a practice computer program go to a real-life setting from that of a practice one

Goals: (1) The objectives to be met or (2) an expected achievement of an employee based on the role's job description, which is evaluated during the review process

Graphical method: The use of graphs to represent data

Gross domestic product (GDP): The value of all goods and services produced in a given period

Gross margin: The amount of money left over from a sale of a product after the COGS are subtracted (synonymous with *gross profits*)

Gross profits: The amount of money left over from a sale of a product after the COGS are subtracted (synonymous with *gross margin*)

H

Hardware: The physical components of a computer and its systems such as a monitor

Health information exchange (HIE): The secure and compatible sharing of health-related information between many different entities including clinics, hospitals, health organizations, and government bodies

Health Insurance Portability and Accountability Act (HIPAA): The Federal law that restricts access to an individual's medical information

Home-equity loan: A loan that can be considered as a second mortgage where the equity of an individual's home is used to obtain a loan that can be used for other immediate needs or to pay off another loan with a higher interest rate

Honor: A quality of behaving in a manner consistent with the highest moral code

Horizontal leadership: A leadership structure where direction is given and information is shared in a side-to-side direction as authority is more spread out over the organization

Human nature: The innate qualities and behaviors of a human being

Human resources: (1) a department within a company that hires, trains, reviews, and terminates employees (denoted as "Human Resources" with capitalized letters or "HR") or (2) the actual human beings that serve as employees (denoted as "human resources" with lower case letters)

Hypertext markup language (HTML): A particular type of coding used in website design that does not change in layout despite a change in display

Hypothesis: A proposed explanation of observations based on limited information

I

Idle time: An inefficient or wasted period of time in a process when available resources can do work but do not have the necessary materials to complete the step

Import: A good produced outside of a nation but sold within it

Incentive: A bonus for achieving a goal

Income: The amount of revenue left over after all costs and expenses are accounted (synonymous with *profit, bottom line,* and *earnings*)

Income statement: A financial statement for a company that describes and calculates its profitability through profits and losses (synonymous with *profit & loss statement*)

Independent variable: A variable where its value does not rely on the value of another variable

Indirect report: A type of reporting in an organization where layers of intermediate reporting exist between individuals

Individual Retirement Account (IRA): A retirement plan that allows an individual to contribute a fixed amount of income every year that can also be tax-deductible depending on certain plans

Inflation: An effect of decreasing the purchasing power of money or an increase in prices overall

Influence: The process of affecting the behavior and thoughts of others

Information technology (IT): The discipline of how information is stored, used, and communicated through the use of computers as its most common vehicle

Intangible assets: The set of assets owned by a company that have value but are not readily measured

Integrity: The ability to behave in a manner consistent with an individual's values and morals

Interest: A financial operation used to describe the extra obligation incurred by borrowing a certain amount of money

Interest rate: The rate at which interest accrues

Interests: The underlying reasons the various sides have each issue

Interface: A method of connection that can take the form of devices or programs

Internal environment: The happenings and atmosphere inside an organization

Internal marketing: Marketing to those within an organization

Internal rate of return (IRR): A method of evaluating investments by expressing how efficiently the money can be utilized

Inventory: The sum of all final products ready for sale along with any available raw materials

Issues: The points of discussion that need to be addressed and agreed upon

J

Job description (JD): A formal description for a position in an organization that provides specifics about its responsibilities and expectations

Job enlargement: An action taken to increase the task load for an employee

Job enrichment: The process of enabling job enlargement for an employee along with the addition of autonomy to perform those required tasks

Job shadowing: The process in which one employee attempts to gain an understanding and perspective of another position by observing other employees in that role

L

Landing page: The page on a company's website where traffic from other sites is directed to start

Lateral communication: An organizational communication style where information is transferred side-to-side in a hierarchy

Law of demand: The idea that as prices for a good increase then the quantity demanded decreases

Law of diminishing return: The concept where the value created for each additional unit output decreases over time

Law of supply: The idea that as prices for a good increase then the quantity supplied increases

Lead time: A quantity of time needed before a required step or process can be initiated

Leader: A person that provides leadership

Leadership: The ability to guide and provide influence to others in both an individual and group setting

Ledger: A company's collection of financial accounts

Leverage: The use of credit from lenders to create profits

Liability: An obligation that a company owes

Life insurance: An insurance plan that pays money to the beneficiaries of an individual in the event of death

Limited Liability Partnership (LLP): A business structure in which more than one person runs a company but are only held to have liability to the degree in which each has invested in the group

Line balancing: A strategy in which certain steps in process are combined or separated to decrease individual idle time by matching the time through the bottleneck step

Line of credit: A form of financing that behaves like a short-term loan from a bank to a company

Liquidity: A description of how easy an asset can be converted to cash

Local hosting: The situation where the location of a company's server used for EHR is physically onsite

Log-rolling: The exchange of smaller agreements on certain issues to achieve a larger agreement based on each side's priorities

Logistics: The planning, managing, and executing of each step in a process

Long-term debt: The amount owed in loans that do not need to be paid within the year

Loss: The situation when costs and expenses exceed net sales

Loyalty: A degree of allegiance where an individual maintains commitment despite external forces

M

Macroeconomics: The study of how resources are used throughout an entire economy

Malware: A malicious software such as a computer virus

Manager: (1) A person that fills a role designated by a company that controls the activities of a group of employees or (2) an employee that governs the overall priorities of those working under him or her

Managerial position: A role in an organization where an employee supervises and manages the activities of those staff members directed to perform duties

Mann-Whitney U test: A non-parametric statistic used to determine if 2 sample means from a population are equal or not

Marginal cost: The extra cost when creating another unit of output

Marginal tax rate: The financial implication where the amount of tax an individual pays varies because the rate increases with additional income generated beyond certain threshold limits

Market economy: The economy created when many different firms and households interact for goods and services in a marketplace

Market expansion: The process in which a company attempts to find new segments of consumers

Market research: A process to understand the market space based on historical evaluation along with present-day surveys

Market segmentation strategy: The process of breaking down a market and its consumers into a smaller yet more homogenous group at which advertisement is directed

Market share: The percentage representation of a company's product or service penetrance in a given market

Marketing: The management process of promoting and selling products and services

Marketing plan: The collection of thoughts and processes used by a company to promote and sell its products and services

Marketing strategy: A section of the marketing plan that delineates the process of how a company's advertising will be performed

Maturity: The length or point in time when payment is due

Mean: A method to calculate an average of a data set by adding the values of the data points and dividing by the number of data points

Meaningful use (MU): The process of using EHR to improve the quality of patient care where specific measures are taken to calculate metrics that are used to receive Medicare funds

Median: A method to calculate an average of a data set by sequencing the data points in numerical order and then picking the number in the middle of the group

Medicare Access and CHIP Reauthorization Act (MACRA): A pay-for-performance government program to replace the current Medicare reimbursement schedule that is intended to focus on quality, value, and accountability through the use of a merit-based incentive payment system

Mentorship: A process where an experienced individual passes along knowledge and provides guidance with the goal of developing another person

Merger: The business process where 2 companies join together

Mergers and acquisitions (M&A): The commonly used phrase to encompass the activities involving mergers and acquisitions

Merit-Based Incentive Payment System (MIPS): A system derived from a collection of PQRS, VBM, and EHR based on MACRA

Metrics: A measure in which output is evaluated

Microeconomics: The study of how individual units or groups make use of resources and their interaction in markets

Milestones: The long-term goals attempted to be accomplished with the aid of negotiations

Mission statement: A statement that represents the purpose and values of a group or organization

Mode: A method to calculate an average of a data set by selecting the value that appears the most

Model: The act of exemplifying a quality, behavior, or action

Monopolies: A situation when one seller can supply all the demand of a market at lower costs than all competitors

Mortgage: The process of charging a piece of property to a creditor under the premise that the control of the property will be turned over to the debtor when payment for it is completed

Motivation: The act of providing encouragement to another person to achieve a goal

Multitasking: The ability to properly perform many duties at one time

Mutual fund: An investment program where a combination of various stocks, bonds, and securities (portfolio) is run by a professional company on behalf of its investors

N

Negative amortization: A situation where the repayment on a loan does not cover the cost of the interest and results in an increase in the principal balance over time

Negative cash flow: The state of a company where there is less cash available at the end than at the beginning, as described by the cash flow statement

Negative reinforcement: The use of giving penalties to employees who do not demonstrate the desired behavior in an organization

Negotiation grid: A preparatory guide created to identify and develop key topics that enables the use of thoughtful tactics to strategically maximize results in a negotiation

Negotiations: The art of deal-making

Net fixed assets: The resultant of subtracting accumulated depreciation from the cost of fixed assets

Net present value (NPV): A calculation used in evaluating investments to determine the PV based on the future value that is discounted

Net sales: The amount that will be collected from a sale minus any discounts provided to the customer to entice the purchase (synonymous with revenue and top line)

Network: The resulting aggregate from a set of interconnected computers and their systems

Noncurrent assets: The set of assets that are not sold routinely and, therefore, are not converted to cash

Non-parametric statistics: Statistics where assumptions to the population distribution cannot be made and the number of parameters can change

Non–value-added (NVA): A wasted expenditure of a resource during a process that does not increase the value of the product or service

Normal distribution: A traditional or Bell spread of a distribution

Normative commitment: An employee's decision to remain with a company based on a feeling of obligation

Null hypothesis (H_0): A hypothesis that the observations noted have occurred by chance events

Numerical method: The use of numbers to represent data

O

Offer: A process in which a prospective employee is given the option to accept the open position in question

Offline: The status of not being connected to another computer or network

Oligopolies: A situation when a few sellers can supply all the demand of a market at lower costs than other competitors

Online: The status of being connected to another computer or network

Online advertising: The use of the Internet to promote a company's products and services

Open-ended question: A style of question where answers invite detailed responses

Operating expenses: A collective group of expenses incurred by a company to provide ancillary support that help generate sales; and these expenses include Sales & Marketing, Research & Development (R&D), and General & Administrative (G&A) (synonymous with SG&A).

Operations: A discipline of business that focuses on the creation, utilization, and improvement of processes in a company

Operations cash: The amount of money generated by cash distributions subtracted from cash receipts

Operations income: The income left over after accounting for all the costs and expenses from the net sales, which is represented by subtracting SG&A from the gross profits

Opportunity cost: A cost given up in the pursuit of creating an output

Opt-in: A method of consumer recruitment where the consumer elects to be included

Opt-out: A method of consumer recruitment where the consumer elects to be excluded

Organizational behavior (OB): The study of how individuals and groups behave and interact with another in an organization

Organizational chart: A diagram where reporting lines are used to illustrate the roles of each individual and their relationship to one another

Organizational framework: The manner in which a company is organized into its structure

Outsourcing: The use of an outside entity to provide a necessary a step or an entire process in operations

Overhead: The cost that is incurred to make a good or provide a service that cannot be directly attributed to the material and labor for that good or service

P

P value: A calculated value of probability typically used in hypothesis testing to quantify the likelihood of an event or its extreme occurring when the null hypothesis is correct

Pages per session: The number of pages viewed by a user on a website

Parametric statistics: Statistics that have a fixed number of parameters that assume the sample from the population follows a probably distribution

Parties: The different sides that are involved in the negotiations

Patent: The legal right of an owner for a design

Patient portal: An electronic platform through which patients, healthcare providers, and their staff can communicate

Pay-per-click (PPC) advertising: A method of online advertisement where every time a viewer clicks on a company's advisement, there is a charge to the company

Pension: A benefit plan given to employees by a company that provides monthly income during retirement based on how long the employee was with the company and what he or she was earning

Percentile: A measure in statistics in which a given percentage of data points fall below or above a certain value

Performance: A description of how well an investment portfolio grew in value over a period of time

Performance efficiency: The effectiveness of an employee's performance relative to a performance standard

Performance rating: The scoring of an employee's performance

Performance standard: A metric used to evaluate employee performance that represents the level of expected achievement

Permutations: The number of ways objects from a set can be grouped together where the order does matter

Personal construct: The way in which an individual sees, interprets, and interacts with the world

Personal finance: The study of an individual's management of money

Personal health record (PHR): A copy of a patient's medical chart, in either electronic or physical form, that is held by the patient

Physician Quality Report System (PQRS): A method to report patient-care quality metrics to Medicare

Population: A set that has all the data points of a group

Positive cash flow: The state of a company where there is more cash available at the end than at the beginning, as described by the cash flow statement

Positive reinforcement: The use of giving beneficial rewards to employees who demonstrate the desired behavior in an organization

Power: The degree to which an individual can exude control over others

Preferred stock: An advanced type of stock where owners are given special considerations during times of dividend distribution or asset allocation for cases of liquidation

Prepaid expenses: The expenses that have been paid already but have not been used

Present value (PV): The current value of money

Price elastic: The condition where there is much change in the amount of a product demanded when there is change in the price

Price elasticity: The amount of responsiveness for a product supplied or demanded based on changes of the price

Price inelastic: The condition where there is no change in the amount of a product demanded when there is a change in the price

Price-to-earnings (P/E) ratio: A financial calculation that relates the price of a stock to the net income earned by a firm

Prime rate: The lowest rate of interest that can be given on loan that is generally held for those with the best credit and least risk to default

Principal: The amount of money borrowed in a loan that still needs to be repaid in addition to the accumulating interest after a payment is made

Print advertising: The use of hardcopy materials to promote a company's products and services

Priorities: The organized list of interests based on a decreasing order of importance

Prioritizing: The ability to order tasks in a fashion in order to first address those with most importance

Privacy: The condition of keeping secret or private (synonymous with *confidentiality*)

Private equity firms: Organizations that are backed by private, and not public, funding used to invest in business opportunities

Pro forma: A model of expected future performance based on historical data and projections that is formatted using the same guidelines as current financial statements

Probability: A measurement in statistics to describe the odds of an event occurring

Process: The cumulative step-by-step procedure of creating a good or providing a service

Process map: A description explaining the relationship of steps in a process

Product line: A group of associated products or services

Product portfolio: The collection of products and services provided by a company

Productivity: The effectiveness of an employee to successfully complete assigned tasks

Profit: The amount of revenue left over after all costs and expenses are accounted (synonymous with *earnings, income,* and *bottom line*)

Profit & loss (P&L) statement: A financial statement for a company that describes and calculates its profitability through profits and losses (synonymous with *income statement*)

Profit margin: A calculation determined by how much of the profit from a sale exceeds its costs

Profitability ratios: A set of financial calculations that describes profitability based on financial markers

Public relations (PR) firms: Companies that manage the outward image of a company and its associated products and services

Pull power: The ability of a marketing activity to draw consumers toward a company for its products and services

Q

Quality assurance: The ability to provide a certain level quality for a product or service

Queue: A line created at a step in a process waiting to proceed forward

R

Radio advertising: The use of radio to promote a company's products and services

Range: A description of a data set that is defined by its extreme values

Recession: A period of time when there is a reduction in the economy usually associated with a decline in gross domestic product

Reference check: A review of a potential employee's references listed on a job application for accuracy and validity

Refinancing: A financial process where an individual obtains a new mortgage with a lower interest rate to pay off his or her currently higher interest rate mortgage

Regression: The relationship of one dependent variable relative to changes with independent variables

Regression analysis: A model in statistics to estimate the relationships of 2 variables

Reinforcement theory: A method of employee thinking that alters the employees behavioral actions based on perceived consequences

Relationship-oriented behavior: A style of decision making that focuses on relationship building

Remote access: The ability to gain entry to a computer and its programs from a distant site or terminal

Remote hosting: The situation where the location of a company's server used for EHR is located elsewhere and made functional through the use of a secure software application

Reservation point: The absolute minimum that each side will accept on an issue that will allow for an agreed upon result

Responsive design: A design structure of a website and its layout to keep it flexible depending on the display used by the consumer

Resume: The experience, training, and skill set of a perspective employee applying for a position

Retained earnings: The amount of profits left behind that are not given as dividends to shareholders

Retargeting: A method of remarketing used online when a consumer that has visited a website is shown an advertisement of a company's product or service later on in the consumer's browsing

Return on investment (ROI): A calculation used to quantify the relationship between the creation of profits and payment of costs for an investment

Revenue: The amount that will be collected from a sale minus any discounts provided to the customer to entice the purchase (synonymous with *net sales* and *top line*)

Revenue cycle manager: The individual within a company that oversees the process (revenue cycle management or RCM) that tracks the payments from patients in a healthcare system from the moment of an encounter presentation until the balance is posted and paid

Reverse mortgage: A financial process where a lender will pay a homeowner on a scheduled basis with cash in exchange for taking equity from the homeowner's house

Risk management: A process used to mitigate legal risk of an organization when possible issues may arise

S

S Corporation: A business structure where the corporation is treated like a partnership, but income is passed through to shareholders and taxed only once

Sales, general, and administrative expenses (SG&A): A collective group of expenses incurred by a company to provide ancillary support that help generate sales. These expenses include sales & marketing, research & development, and general & administrative (synonymous with *operating expenses*)

Sales position: A role in an organization where an employee is part of the sales force

Sample: A set that has a fraction of all the data points of a group

Scapegoat: An action where the blame of a negative outcome or situation is placed on one or a few individuals that bares the responsibility for the undesired result

Scarcity: The condition that resources are limited in nature

Search engine: A program that identifies appropriate sites from a database given the set of keywords entered

Search engine optimization (SEO): The methods used to improve the ranking of a website when a search engine is used

Securities and Exchange Commission (SEC): The US government agency in charge of protecting investors from malpractice by companies, brokers, and advisors

Self-directed work team: A group of individuals that by themselves have the ability to identify, assess, plan, and execute actions when faced with problems

Session users: The number of unique viewers of a website

Shareholders' equity: A representation of value held by an owner in a company that is determined by the sum of capital stock and retained earnings

Shortage: A condition when the amount of supply available is less than its demand

Site map: A list of the different pages that a user can access on a website

Situation: The current problem(s) that need to be addressed in the negotiation

Skew distribution: A loop-sidedness of a distribution

Skill-based pay method: A merit-based system that rewards employees that grow their skill set and meet certain milestones in development

Skills: The composition of an employee's innate and learned abilities

Social media: The various methods used for the purpose of social networking

Social networking: The use of social media to create and communicate content that is shared with others that are connected to the creator

Socialization: The way an organization is run by social rules of conduct and behavior

Software: The nonphysical components of a computer and its systems such as a computer program

Sole proprietorship: A business structure where the individual and his or her company are treated like a single entity with regard to taxes and liability

Solid line: A type of line used in organizational charts denoting authority from a supervisor to a subordinate

Stakeholders: Represents the collection of individuals that has an interest in the outcome of the negotiation even if they are not physically present

Standard deviation: A description of a data set that expresses the degree to which there is dispersion of the set's values

Statistics: The study of the collection and analysis of data

Stereotype: The attribution of certain qualities to another person based on their group membership, such as gender or race

Stock: A representation of ownership in a corporation

Stocks: The shares sold by a company to raise funds

Strategies: The purposeful use of actions to achieve a goal

Strengths, Weaknesses, Opportunities, and Threats (SWOT) Analysis: A structured form of analysis to better understand the current positioning of an individual or company in its appropriate competitive landscape

Substitutes: A relationship between 2 products where an increase in the price of one leads to a decrease in the demand for the other

Succession training: A process in which the needed skill set of a particular position is passed from a superior to a lower-level employee with the goal of one day assuming the higher role

Suitability: The fit of an employee's ability to a particular need or task for a position in an organization

Sunk cost: A cost that has already occurred and cannot be recouped

Superuser: An individual user that has restricted control to manage and administer a system

Supervisor: An employee that directly oversees the tasks and performance of the individuals below him or her

Surplus: A condition when the amount of a supply available is greater than its demand

T

T-score: Standardized scores used in statistics

T-test: A statistical test that assesses if 2 sets of data are significantly different from each other

Tactics: The tasks that are completed to produce an action

Takt time: The actual cycle time or the inverse of throughput

Target: The goal each side has for the issues

Target audience: The specific consumer base that a marketing campaign is attempting to convert over to become customers of a company

Task-oriented behavior: A style of decision making that focuses on getting objectives met

Task list: A to-do list commonly seen in EHR where the creator of the list can be the individual user of the system or those connected to the user

Taxes payable: The amount of income tax a practice owes the government

Team-building techniques: Various methods used to initiate, develop, and maintain a team-oriented approach

Teamwork: The process where a group of individuals work together as a cohesive unit to achieve goals

Technical support: The service to help users with computer and associated systems issues

Television advertising: The use of television to promote a company's products and services

Termination: The process where an employee is relieved of his or her duties in an organization because of a particular reason (for cause termination) or without one (without cause termination)

Testimonials: Customer review statements about a company's products and services

Throughput: The amount of output a process can achieve in a set period of time

Time management: The ability to efficiently allot the limited resource of time to accomplish goals

Top line: The amount that will be collected from a sale minus any discounts provided to the customer to entice the purchase (synonymous with *net sales* and *revenue*)

Total cost: The value of all costs incurred to create a given output

Trademark: A legally registered word or symbol that represents a company or product

Trainer: A qualified user of a system that educates those using it

Transferable skills: A set of skills that can be used over a wide range of positions with differing job descriptions

Turnover: The percentage of employees that depart and are replaced relative to the number of total employees in an organization

U

Underwriting: The procedure in which a company evaluates the risk of an individual to file a claim that can either determine rates or even refuse an application

Upgrades: The addition of new software or hardware to update the pre-existing ones

Upward communication: An organizational communication style where information is transferred from the bottom of a hierarchy to the top

URL: A website's address

Utilization: A metric that describes how efficiently a process is being used and defined as the ratio of throughput over capacity

V

Value-added (VA): An expenditure of a resource during a process that increases the value of the product or service

Value-based payment modifier (VBM): A method to provide different payment to physicians based on the quality compared to the cost of that care

Values: The amount of worth someone places on certain things

Variability: An inconsistent or unpredictable quality of something

Variable cost: A cost that does vary depending on the output quantity created

Variance: A description of a data set that is the mean of the squared distances for each point to the population's mean

Vertical leadership: A leadership structure where leaders are positioned at the top of a hierarchical-based organization with the authority to give direction while those at the bottom follow orders and provide information upward

View-through rate (VTR): The percentage of consumers that view a company's ad and visit the company's website soon after

Virus: A type of computer malware that replicates and integrates into a computer and its system's programs and files

Vision statement: A statement that describes the direction and goals of a group or organization

Vlog: A video blog

W

Wait time: The time spent at a step in a process waiting to proceed forward

Waste: An inefficient use of valued resource

Web identity: The summation of everything on the Internet that mentions and relates to a company along with its products and services

Website: The location of an entity on the Internet that connects to various associated pages

Website analytics: The process of obtaining, measuring, and analyzing data from the use of a website in order to improve its performance and positioning

Website traffic: The movement of users entering and leaving a website

Wellness program: A support system within an organization that focuses on employee well-being, including the issue of burnout

Wilcoxon Signed Rank test: A non-parametric statistic used to test if 2 dependent samples were taken from a population of the same distribution

Will: A formal document that expresses one's desire for how his or her assets will be cared for and allocated along with care for the individual's family

Word of mouth: A method of advertisement that spreads recommendations about a company and its associated products and services directly from one past consumer to a prospective one

Workplace politics: The inner workings and relationships within an organization that influence how it and the employees operate

Other

401(k): A common retirement plan provided by for-profit companies that allow employee contributions to compound over time without taxation, along with the added benefit of being exempt from federal and state taxes

5 Ps: The 5 components of a marketing strategy (product, price, placement, promotion, people)

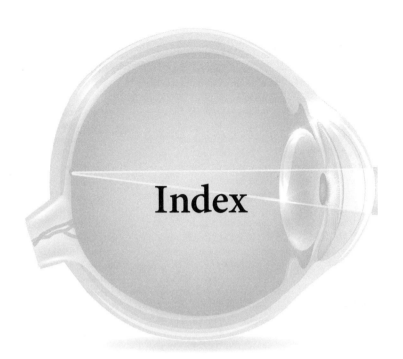

Index